Health and Social Care Theory and Practice:
Values for Care Practice

Health and Social Care Theory and Practice:

Values for Care Practice

Sue Cuthbert and Jan Quallington

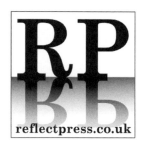

reflectpress.co.uk

First published in 2008

ISBN: 978 1 906052 05 8

British Library Cataloguing in Publication Data
A catalogue record for this book is available from the British Library

Production project management by Deer Park Productions

Typeset by PDQ Typesetting

Cover design by Oxmed

Printed and bound by Cromwell Press Ltd, Trowbridge, Wiltshire

Distributed by BEBC, Albion Close, Parkstone, Poole, Dorset BH12 3LL

Published by Reflect Press Ltd
11 Attwyll Avenue
Exeter
Devon, EX2 5HN
UK
01392 204400
www.reflectpress.com

Contents

Health and Social Care Series

Series Editors: Sue Cuthbert, Jan Quallington and Elaine Donnelly – all at the University of Worcester

This series of textbooks is aimed at students on Health and Social Care Foundation Degree programmes in FE and HE institutions. However, the books also provide short introductions to key topics for Common Foundation Programme modules and will be suitable for first-year undergraduate courses in a variety of Health and Social Care subject areas. Books in the series will also be useful for those returning to practice and for overseas nursing students. The series includes three types of textbook:

Knowledge and Skills books;
Theory and Practice books;
Specialist books that cover specific professions, topics and issues.

All titles in the series will address the common elements articulated in relevant sector skill frameworks such as, for example, Skills for Care, Skills for Health, the NHS Knowledge and Skills Framework and the Code of Practice for Social Care Workers.

Other titles in the series include:

An Introduction to the Principles and Practice of Care by Peter Unwin
ISBN: 978 1 906052 03 4 (publication due summer 2008)

Understanding Research and Evidence-based Practice by Bruce Lindsay
ISBN: 978 1 906052 01 0

Communication and Interpersonal Skills by Elaine Donnelly and Lindsey Neville
ISBN: 978 1 906052 06 5

Safe and Clean Care: Infection Prevention and Control for Health and Social Care Students by Tina Tilmouth with Simon Tilmouth
ISBN: 978 1 906052 08 9 (publication due summer 2008)

Work-based Learning and Practice Placement: A Textbook for Health and Social Care Edited by Graham Brotherton and Steven Parker
ISBN: 978 1 906052 12 6 (publication due summer 2008)

Essential Study Skills for Health and Social Care Edited by Marjorie Lloyd and Peggy Murphy
ISBN: 978 1 906052 14 0 (publication due summer 2008)

Foreword

The authors of this book, who are both involved in the teaching of ethics and values across a broad range of courses, have developed an introductory text that explores values as a central consideration in care practice. When we first talked about writing this book we felt it represented an opportunity to write a book to support our teaching and to help students to explore the value base of health and social care work. We envisaged that our readers would all be students new to the formal study of health and social care and that they would be involved in working across a wide range of health and social care settings and with a broad mix of people. This book is also designed to be a useful study guide and reference text for teachers working on and developing new modules or courses within the same field of study as ourselves.

This foundation text is one of a series of texts that are designed to introduce the core elements of health and social care. The textbooks also provide the opportunity for students to develop and apply their learning within their specific practice context, with a particular emphasis on integrating theory and practice and learning through reflective activity.

WHO IS THIS BOOK AIMED AT?

The book will be suitable for a wide range of students who aspire to develop and reflect on their knowledge, skills and attitudes in the world of contemporary health and care. The teaching team at the University of Worcester are working collaboratively to offer an innovative programme of foundation studies for developing professionals such as nurses and paramedics and social care workers, and for the emerging roles of assistant practitioners and support workers in health and social care. This book is designed to support the shared learning experiences of these practitioners in exploring the value base of the health and social care sectors. An essential element of health and social care education programmes is work-based learning. Students must be able to apply their learning within their own, specific, vocational context. Therefore, applying theory to practice in work-based learning environments is a central theme in the book. This book will utilise examples drawn from a range of care settings and different client groups.

HOW TO USE THIS BOOK

The book includes a range of strategies designed to enhance your learning and these are illustrated by the different types of activities that are used. Spending time thinking and completing these activities will result in a deeper understanding of the values and issues discussed.

Key themes

The key themes listed at the beginning of each chapter indicate the main points that are addressed in that chapter. You will find side headings indicating where each of the key themes is addressed within the chapter.

Reading activity

There are texts that you will need to read that cannot be included as part of this book, such as documents published by the government. These texts will be indicated in the reading activity boxes. You will be given the details of the document and a web address from which you can download it.

Reflection

The most common type of activity that you will be asked to undertake is reflection. Some of these activities are very short and some can be carried out over a few days. You might be asked to make a few short notes as part of the reflection.

Writing activity

In a writing activity you will be asked to either make extensive notes or write a few pages on a subject. These activities might take a comparatively short time or they may extend over a few days.

Discussion activity

Discussion activities provide an opportunity for you to explore an issue from different perspectives. You can do these in a group setting or using a web-based discussion facility.

Question

A question activity is a short activity that directs you to think about a specific issue and to respond with an answer.

Imaginative exercise

An imaginative exercise requires you to think about a hypothetical situation. It can be undertaken as a solitary exercise on your own or you can do this in discussion with others.

Case study

A case study is a slightly more in-depth activity and directs you to explore some of the more complex and complicated issues that arise when caring for others.

AUTHOR BIOGRAPHIES

Sue Cuthbert

Sue Cuthbert is a Principal Lecturer in the Institute of Health, Social Care and Psychology at the University of Worcester. She qualified as a Registered General Nurse and has practised in care of the older adult and women's health settings. She moved into nurse education in 1987 and has most recently led curriculum development for and taught on a range of courses in health and social care, from foundation degree through to masters level. Her teaching and academic research interests are predominantly focused on ethics and values in health and social care, with a particular emphasis on ethical issues at the beginning of life, rights to health care, resource allocation, reproductive choice and access to infertility treatment. Sue is currently undertaking doctoral research related to autonomy and informed choice in antenatal decisions at Keele University.

Jan Quallington

Jan Quallington is a Principal Lecturer in the Institute of Health, Social Care and Psychology at the University of Worcester. She qualified as a State Registered Nurse and practised in acute medicine and intensive therapy units. She moved into higher education in 1986 and has taught across a range of professional and non-professional programmes from foundation degree to masters programmes. Her current role is the responsibility for quality assurance and enhancement and curriculum development across the Institute of Health, Social Care and Psychology. Her academic interests are in applying ethics and values to health and social care contexts, with a particular interest in values as they are played out in policy and consequently practice. Jan is undertaking doctoral research on public involvement in health care planning.

Introduction

VALUES AND CARE

Values are a fundamental component of the provision, practice and delivery of health and social care. The development of personal and professional values is influenced by a number of factors and the values held by practitioners and their professional groups can lead to competing demands and duties that make decision-making complex.

In this book, readers will be encouraged to critically analyse their personal value base and those values that underpin health and social care work. The reader will explore values in general and reflect on how these are articulated in codes of practice and applied in practice. The text will use activities and case studies to enable the reader to reflect on the relevance of values in care practice and to apply theory in your practice.

Values are inescapable and an integral feature of care practice. Caring is not and should not be just a practical activity but is a quality of character which involves genuine concern for the health, welfare and well-being of the individuals receiving care. Although not universally true, many of the individuals receiving care are likely to experience vulnerability; by virtue of illness, age, disability, pain or loss of confidence. Care is essentially an interpersonal activity so, therefore, delivering care requires not only knowledge and skills but a caring attitude that is value-based. Although competence, efficiency and effectiveness are important components of good care they are not sufficient in themselves; what matters most is not just what you do but how you do it. The verb 'to care' implies not merely a functional activity (as, for example, the verb 'to run' does); it also implies an activity that has a qualitative dimension. This dimension says something about the way in which caring is carried out. The verb 'to care' can be defined by using phrases such as: 'to be concerned about', 'to be watchful of', 'to have a liking for' and 'to pay close attention to'. Caring is not a purely practical task that needs to be completed as efficiently as possible, but implies that the completion of the activity is undertaken with a particular attitude. Values are particular kinds of beliefs that are concerned with the worth of an idea or behaviour and are important in guiding our actions, our judgements, our behaviour and our attitudes to others. Values play an essential role in articulating the standards and manner for the delivery of care. The values explored in this text are those that dominate care in modern, Western societies.

VALUES AND MORALS

The very nature of health or social care work is that it is practical; it involves doing as well as understanding. You will need to know that something is the case, such as a fact of law or of anatomy and physiology, as well as knowing how to do something, such as a practical skill. The factual or knowledge base to perform the skills associated with care practice can be wide-ranging, dependent upon your area of practice and level of expertise. For example, you may need to know how to perform urinalysis, how to safely move an immobile patient, how to listen effectively, how to apply a dressing to a wound, how to organise and run a group activity with service users, how to communicate with a person with hearing loss. You will learn the facts associated with 'knowing that' and 'knowing how' through teaching and through practice. However, there is another essential component to understanding in health and social care that has a significant influence on what you do and how you practise, and that is the moral dimension of practice.

Your personal beliefs and attitudes regarding the way you should behave towards others, why you should act in a particular way and what you think is the right or wrong thing to do are heavily influenced by your moral understanding and your values. Values are different to factual knowledge because they are harder to quantify, standardise or provide evidence for. However, their impact on the care relationship is fundamental. Put simply, values are what we believe is worthy or valuable and our values guide our actions, our judgements, our behaviour and our attitudes to others.

The concept of values may encompass a range of meanings and be understood in different ways and contexts, not all of which will be directly associated with morality. A value may describe an emotional disposition towards a person, object or idea; may be something we recognise as good or worthwhile; or reflect a personal belief or attitude about the truth, beauty or worth of a thought, object or behaviour (Pattison, 2004, pp.5–6). For example, when asked the value you attribute to a picture, you could respond by simply telling me how much it cost, you could talk about the reputation of the artist, you could say that it is beautiful and that you love it or you could tell me that it cost very little but it is priceless to you because of its sentimental value in reminding you of a special relationship. Values may be used to describe the worth, importance or

usefulness of something to someone. Seedhouse (1998, pp. 78–9) identifies a number of categories of things we may attribute value to,
including:

- physical objects – for example, your car or your house;
- aesthetic qualities such as beauty, for example, works of art, beautiful
  gardens, etc.;
- intangibles such as friendships, creativity, etc.;
- principles or rules of behaviour, like truth-telling, sanctity of life, etc.;
- ideologies, for example, liberalism.

Pattison (2004, pp. 3–5) outlines a number of synonyms used either in
conjunction with, or instead of, the language of values.

- Preferences, desires and choices – from the economic domain, i e.
  people value or confer worth on what they prefer, desire or choose
  (and are prepared to pay for).
- Attitudes and beliefs – from the psychological domain, i.e. what people
  are attitudinally predisposed to or believe in is what they value and can
  be discerned by watching their behaviour, such as, for example, voting
  for a particular political party.
- Social norms, assumptions, expectations, judgements and prejudices –
  the sociological domain, i.e. what holds people together in groups so
  that society is coherent and individual behaviour is predictable; shared
  views of what is good or bad, desirable and undesirable.
- Standards, visions and goals – the domain of management and governance. Standards are norms of what is expected and required and define
  sufficient value; visions provide a set of ideal standards to which people
  can aspire; goals are the intermediate specific value targets which must
  be reached.
- Morals, principles and commitments – the domain of morality and
  ethics. Morals are precepts or habits that aim to attain what is good
  and desirable, i.e. what is valued. Principles aim to ensure certain values
  are realised. Commitments are a form of consent to a set of values.

The definition of value is therefore multifaceted and complex. We will
draw on all of the different expressions of values listed above. However,
what is commonly meant when discussing values in health and social care
(and is of main concern here) are the moral beliefs, principles or rules of
conduct that guide our social interactions and human relationships.
Individuals generally hold personal beliefs and values that are important
to them and that influence their actions and behaviours towards others.

WHERE DO BELIEFS AND VALUES COME FROM?

Much of our development of values and moral reasoning takes place during childhood and adolescence. However, these values may not be consciously selected or subjected to any scrutiny but are rather acquired from family and early socialisation or assimilated from cultural norms in education and play. Our development of moral knowledge is influenced by a number of factors and these include our parents and siblings, peer groups, culture, personality, education, religion and some form of ideology. Values are often subjective and can also be relative to the individual and their circumstances, culture, relationships and experiences. So, although our basic moral foundations of right and wrong, good and bad, what we ought or ought not to do are laid down in childhood, our values are not static and will inevitably be influenced by our experiences throughout life, including those values acquired from professional codes and working practices. Individuals may even reprioritise their values several times in the same day as they attempt to fit in with group norms or they will reprioritise their values at different stages of life or in response to various experiences. Yet, there may also be some values that remain unchanged, that you are not willing to compromise and would take risks to defend.

Individuals are confronted with moral issues every day of their lives (and these are not all to do with health or care). Requests for donations to charities, whether or not you recycle your rubbish, what you do when you are given too much change at the checkout, when your friend tells you about her affair with a colleague and asks you not to tell her husband. Many everyday circumstances and decisions have a moral component so it should not be surprising that morality pervades your role and your decision-making as a practitioner in health or social care. Good, effective communication and interpersonal skills are essential throughout care practice; both in your work with patients, services users, clients, their families and carers and with other formal carers and professionals across a range of settings (see Donnelly and Neville, 2008). What is also important is the moral dimension that comes into your decisions about how and what to communicate and a genuine caring attitude, which will inevitably be influenced by your personal value position.

Reflection

1. Before you read the rest of this book it would be useful for you to reflect on your personal values. Identify your core values: those beliefs that you hold that you would not be willing to compromise like, for example, that it is wrong to cause harm to another. Make a list.

2. Now order this list of personal values, placing the one that is most important to you at the top.
3. Once you have 'rank ordered' your values, try to say why each is important to you. It may help to use the stem:

I believe............................because..........................

For example, 'I believe it is wrong to intentionally harm another because life is precious and you should treat others the way you would wish to be treated yourself'.

VALUES AND REFLECTION

You may think that the moral dimension is just a matter of intuition or common sense, and not something that can or needs to be learned. While we all live by some personal value base, we don't always appreciate why we believe the things we do or we may be inconsistent in our values. There are often no clear or right answers, so reflection and further exploration are important elements of value-based study. The reality is that codes of practice identify broad guidelines or principles but cannot tell you exactly how they should be applied in your everyday work or how to resolve issues where values conflict. Equally, you may have found it difficult to verbalise and to provide justification for your key values in the activity above. Yet, at some point, you may be called to account regarding your moral judgements. Great emphasis is placed on reflective practice in personal and professional development in health and social care. However, any critical reflection on your own and others' practice should start from the position of having identified and reflected on your own values. You will no doubt find that many of the things that trouble you (or deserve celebrating) in yours and others practice are those that challenge or concur with your personal value position. Having identified and prioritised your core values will help you to critically analyse issues in practice as well as helping to provide reasons or justifications for your value or moral judgements.

THE RELATIONSHIP BETWEEN PERSONAL AND PROFESSIONAL VALUES

Moral values can be observed on at least three different but interrelated dimensions: at the level of you as an individual (your moral integrity and being true to yourself), in your direct interactions with others (personal encounters and relationships) and at a wider societal level, e.g. justice and fairness of groups or majorities. Although this book is chiefly aimed at exploring and reflecting on your personal values and how these influence your direct interactions with individuals in your care, the wider social morality inevitably influences your practice too. For example, the way in which resources are distributed in health and social care and whether this is done fairly and justly will impact on your care decisions with individuals, even though you may feel that this is far removed from your realm of influence.

Groups of practitioners often hold or aspire to collective beliefs and common value positions concerning the ways they should behave and their duties and obligations to service users and patients. It may be that the kinds of people attracted to working in care roles come with some similarities in values and beliefs. For professional groups, the profession's collective value position may be defined by a particular professional body and described as a set of standards or in a code of conduct or practice. However, all members of the health and care professions share some common values and principles, even if these are described in different ways. For example, social workers talk about anti-discriminatory practice, learning disability nurses about person-centred approaches, whereas adult nurses and midwives may emphasise respect for autonomy and the processes and practices that can help to achieve this. If you look beyond the differences in language you will see that all of these principles and practices are based in the values of respect for persons and humanity. As Banks (2006, p.7) identifies, the term 'values' can be used to describe both the broader beliefs about the nature of a good society, such as a belief in the worth of human dignity, and more specific conduct-guiding principles that promote the belief, such as respect for an individual's autonomy. Our book will talk about values in both of these ways and sets out to identify the values fundamental to health and care practice. In view of the fact that values are so integral to the provision of care, it is not just professional groups that have expressed values for practice. It has been recognised that care workers should be governed by a minimum set of values and, for this reason, the General Social Care Council (GSCC) published the *Code of Practice for Social Care Workers* (GSCC, 2002) to articulate an agreed standard for practice.

Personal and professional values could be viewed as being distinct, in that your personal values may differ from those of another practitioner even though you belong to a specific care group and both observe the same code of practice. For example, your position on the moral status of the fetus and abortion may be very different to that of a colleague and yet you both work as maternity support workers with shared work values which may be influenced, although not bound by, the Nursing and Midwifery Council's (NMC's) *NMC Code of Professional Conduct: Standards for Conduct, Performance and Ethics* (NMC, 2004). Whatever you value in your personal life influences your moral conscience and behaviour and the judgements and decisions you make, which includes those made in your work. Thus, the boundaries between personal and professional work values inevitably become blurred in their origin and influence. Equally, your personal values and principles may also come into conflict with one another, giving rise to moral dilemmas in your own practice. For example, consider your beliefs about lying and truth-telling. Do you always tell the truth or are there occasions when you evade telling the truth or consider a 'little white lie' as being permissible? Do you tell a friend that their new hairstyle looks ridiculous even if they are really pleased with it? When you are under-charged at the checkout by £10, do you point it out to the cashier? What about £1 . . . or 1p? Pattison (2004, pp.7–8) draws the distinction between 'normal' values and 'aspirational' values. What we are often referring to when we talk of values are the norms, rules, habits, expectations and assumptions that are at the heart of society and form the basis of social interaction and relationships. In this way, 'normal values' generally go unnoticed and require little or no justification or active commitment; they simply exist as part of the fabric of society. However, it is when these 'normal' values are challenged that passions rise and people become defensive, hurt and angry. Aspirational values are those that go beyond the norm; they are the goals and visions; beliefs and values that we aspire to and would like to see integrated effectively in our own practice. This book provides the opportunity for you to consider in more depth those values that are fundamental to good care practice.

While our main aim is to focus on values that contribute to good practice, it is important that you appreciate that not all value positions are good or lead to positive or beneficial outcomes for others. It is quite possible for individuals to vehemently defend their 'values' even though they may have disastrous consequences for others or exclude important concerns, such as in cases of extreme fundamentalism which overrides the beliefs and values of others.

BEING A GOOD PRACTITIONER

Although we will talk a lot in this book about the values that influence your duties or obligations to others in your care, it is also important to consider what it is to be a 'good' practitioner. This can be expressed in terms of your moral character or virtues, which incorporate a complex structure of habits, attitudes, beliefs, motives and emotions that encapsulate the positive values to which you aspire and impact on your personal judgements and actions. Beauchamp and Childress (2001, p.30) highlight some of the virtues often associated with health and care practitioners, derived both from social expectations and from standards and ideals internal to practitioner roles. These include:

- compassion;
- empathy;
- sincerity;
- discernment;
- trustworthiness;
- integrity;
- conscientiousness;
- benevolence and non-malevolence (doing good and not harming);
- truthfulness;
- respectfulness.

This list is by no means exhaustive but it starts to identify some of the standards and ideals of moral character important to health and care practice relationships. We might add wisdom (the need for sound judgement to inform practice) and courage (the courage to put your values into practice). It is the practitioner's personal moral qualities that are of prime importance to service users, patients, clients and their families. However, the possession of virtues or good personal qualities by all practitioners cannot be prescribed because it is essential that these are deeply rooted in the person concerned and developed out of personal commitment rather than the requirement of an external authority. As Pattison (2004, p.5) suggests, being a virtuous (or good) practitioner is about more than simply following a set of rules (such as those you find in codes of conduct or practice). However, by adopting and conforming to certain values in the pursuit of particular visions or ends practitioners can become 'habitually virtuous' such that the values, habits and attitudes become second nature and an essential part of the individual's character, both in their everyday life and their practice. It is with this in mind that this text aims to help you to explore the key values that we believe are essential to good care practice. These values are covered in each chapter as follows.

Chapter 1. Rights, equality and anti-discriminatory practice

A focus on rights has been included in this text because values that are articulated and promised by practitioners and expected by service users and carers are often claimed as rights. This chapter will introduce the notion of rights, explore different kinds of rights and specifically reflect on those relevant to care practice. In particular, it will examine the concepts of equality and anti-discrimination and reflect on strategies that can be employed to support and uphold rights in practice.

Chapter 2. Respect and Dignity

We view respect for persons as a fundamental value for everyday social interactions which also underpins the values associated with health and social care practice. This chapter aims to help you to consider what it means to be respectful and to have respect for others. It explores the concepts of respect, respect for persons, personhood, dignity and privacy. The value of respect for persons and dignity is examined and you will reflect on care strategies that promote respect and dignity in your practice.

Chapter 3. Autonomy and the principle of respect for autonomy

Chapter 3 builds on the notion of respect for persons introduced in Chapter 2 by focusing its discussion on the value of autonomy and the principle of respect for autonomy. It highlights the distinction between a person being autonomous and the principle of respect for autonomy. It offers some definitions of personal autonomy and explores in more detail what it means to be autonomous, including the necessary conditions of competence or capacity. Respect for autonomy is often viewed as a primary principle for guiding health and social care practice; however, this should be balanced with consideration of other important values, such as avoiding risk and harm. The notion of paternalism is introduced here but you will explore further the values of 'Protection from harm and promoting independence' in Chapter 5. Respecting autonomy is not just about agreeing with the wishes of others, and you are encouraged to consider strategies for practice that foster autonomy and enable individuals to be autonomous.

Chapter 4. Trust, confidentiality and truth-telling

Trust is said to be at the heart of health and care practice. It is difficult, if not impossible, to form a good therapeutic relationship without an element of trust between the individuals involved, and service users and patients need to be confident that they can trust the practitioners delivering their care to be concerned for their well-being and to act in their best interests. This chapter will explore the value of trust and trustworthiness and help you to recognise the importance of trust in the practitioner/service user relationship, focusing on the examples of confidentiality and truth-telling.

Chapter 5. Protection from harm and promoting independence

Protection from harm and the promotion of independence are central values for care work. These core values arise out of the 'duty of care' that is owed to the service user by anyone who is contracted to protect their interests and to provide a care service. However, it is essential that this is balanced with the requirement to promote independence, which can, at times, cause tension for practitioners. This chapter will consider the duty of care in protecting service users and reflect on the concept of risk, the principles of risk assessment and risk management in the care context. It will explore the value of independence and apply the notion of planned risk-taking to the care context.

Chapter 6. Values, accountability and responsibility

In this book we spend a great deal of time exploring and unpacking the values inherent in health and social care and reflect on how these values can be integrated into practice. The values that underpin care interventions are probably one of the most significant determinants of the quality of the care that a client receives, and understanding them is consequently of enormous importance. The values that are expressed by different groups in the care sector dictate the standards of care that are subsequently developed and that are reflected directly in the care that is then provided to clients. These standards articulate the responsibilities of the practitioner and it is against these that you could be called to account for your practice. This chapter will reflect on care standards that are derived from core values and explore the extent to which practitioners are responsible for the care that they provide and their level of accountability.

Chapter 7. Conclusion – Value-based reflection

This chapter summarises the key points developed in previous chapters in the book and reiterates the central role of values in developing good care practice. However, this chapter points out that understanding values in care and integrating them into practice does not stop with reading a book. Care practitioners will throughout their careers need to revisit and reflect on the values that underpin their own and others' practice. Practitioners will at times be confronted by challenging situations where there is no obvious resolution. With this in mind, this final chapter introduces the concept of 'value-based reflection'. This provides guidance for care practitioners to examine and improve the care that they provide.

DEFINITIONS

It is recognised in this book that people are cared for in a variety of settings by a wide range of practitioners from different organisations (statutory, non-statutory, independent, and voluntary) and both formal and informal carers. For brevity, we will use the term 'practitioner' to refer to any health or social care employee who delivers care in its broadest sense and the term 'carer' refers to both formal and informal carers, including families, relatives and significant others. If we use the term 'professional' it is intended to refer specifically to any registered health or social care practitioner regulated by a professional statutory body. It is harder to identify a single term that best encompasses the notion of service user, patient or client; we will use all of these terms according to what best suits the situation being discussed.

Further reading

Banks, S. (2001) *Ethics and values in social work*. 2nd ed. Houndmills, Basingstoke: Palgrave Macmillan

Jasper, M. (2003) *Foundations in nursing and health care: beginning reflective practice*. Cheltenham: Nelson Thornes

Seedhouse, D. (1998) *Ethics: the heart of health care*. 2nd ed. Chichester: John Wiley & Sons

Chapter 1

Rights, Equality and Anti-discriminatory Practice

Key themes

In this chapter you will:

- be introduced to the notion of rights;

- explore different kinds of rights;

- focus on rights relevant to care practice;

- examine the concepts of equality and anti-discrimination;

- reflect on strategies that can be employed to support and uphold rights in practice.

INTRODUCTION

Beliefs about individual value and respect for others are important considerations in modern, Western, democratic societies. The principle of respect for others suggests that individuals, just because they are individuals, are important. Their importance is not attributed to their role or position in society or their achievements; rather it is because they are a person (this will be explored further in Chapter 2). Being a person in Western societies brings with it certain rights that are not afforded to other species. The acceptance that individuals have rights also means that there are obligations from others to ensure that conditions exist in which rights can be upheld. This chapter will examine what rights recipients of care services should be afforded and seeks to identify how a care worker can help to support these rights. A section on rights has been included in this text on values because values, that are articulated and promised by practitioners, and expected by clients, are often claimed as rights by service users. This is particularly evident in situations when individuals feel that they are not receiving the care to which they believe they are entitled. Thus rights and values are intrinsically connected.

We live in a society in which we enjoy a multitude of rights, many of which are protected in law. In our day-to-day lives we are normally able to ensure that our rights are respected and that we have the opportunity to challenge this when we feel that our rights have been infringed. However, when individuals come into contact with care services their rights may be put at risk. Individuals in receipt of care may be outside their normal environment, which makes them feel that their personal control has been eroded. They may be feeling vulnerable, frail, in pain, frightened, bewildered, confused, out of their depth or simply lacking knowledge of their entitlements. One of the key roles of the care worker is to understand what rights individuals are entitled to, to uphold these in their interactions with others, to challenge infringement of rights and to support individuals to gain and maintain their rights. Seedhouse (1998) asserts that the way that we treat those who are most vulnerable in our society is a reflection of the moral state of that society. That is to say that we should be concerned about the rights of others and, in particular, the rights of those who are most vulnerable. This chapter will introduce the notion of individual rights and will discuss the responsibilities or obligations of practitioners, users and carers in the appropriate fulfilment of rights.

Reflection

1. Can you think of a situation in which you felt that your rights were not respected?
2. How did this make you feel?
3. Can you identify what led to your rights being challenged?
4. On reflection, was the challenge to your rights justified or unjustified?

WHAT ARE RIGHTS?

The endorsement and protection of rights are an important element of democratic societies. Rights and the importance of the protection of rights became firmly embedded in society following the revelations of the mass violation of human rights that occurred during the Second World War. The idea of rights comes from the strongly held belief that individuals are unique and valuable and that they should, therefore, be accorded respect and the privileges that arise from that status. It is claimed that a focus on rights is important because it enables us to address an issue from the point of view of the victim or the vulnerable rather than from the perspective of those in power who traditionally make the rules (Almond, 1991).

Rights, in the twenty-first century, are often interpreted as 'entitlements'. An entitlement is something that I can reasonably expect from another individual, or from society. This may be expressed as a right or a 'valid claim'. It is helpful to see rights in terms of claims because it reminds us that in exercising our rights we are often requiring or claiming that right from someone else. That is, we are requiring someone else to provide something for us. While this chapter will focus mainly on the idea of rights as claims, there are other definitions of rights.

- **Privileges** are something that one is offered which, because they are not an entitlement, can be withdrawn. For example, in an overcrowded train you may be offered the privilege of sitting in the first-class compartment of the train if there are spare seats, even if you only have a second-class ticket. However, this is not a right.
- **Powers** include, for example, the right to determine what happens with your property after your death.
- **Immunities** are protection from the actions of another. For example, sex discrimination legislation protects women from an exploitative employer, who may wish to pay women less than men (Almond, 1991).

Our society affords us a number of rights or valid claims. For example, I have the right to access education up to the age of 18, I have the right to vote once I reach the age of majority, and I have the right to receive free health care. While I have the rights to make these claims, the rights to these things are not without boundaries. Access to free health care is a reasonable, or valid, claim, given that Britain has a National Health Service (NHS), paid for by direct taxation. However, because the NHS is subject to limited resources, my right to receive health care is not unlimited. My right to receive health care must be balanced against the rights of others to receive health care. The conditions of 'valid' and 'reasonable' claims are important in the context of rights. It would not be reasonable for me to claim numerous, unnecessary, plastic surgery operations in an effort to make myself look better, if this was at the expense of someone else's right to claim life-saving treatment. It is, therefore, a valid claim to seek necessary treatment but not to seek unnecessary treatment.

DIFFERENT KINDS OF RIGHTS

Claims, rights or entitlements are sometimes termed 'positive rights'. These rights require society, or another individual, to do something positive in order to fulfil or uphold the rights. For example, my claim for health care can only be realised if society ensures that health care systems exist for me to access health care, and if individuals in those systems fulfil their duty to provide me with the necessary care.

Human rights

These rights have been agreed by the international community as being the rights that any human is entitled to by virtue of them being human. Many societies protect these through the legal system but, when they are challenged, they may also be protected through the international community. For example, the international community may intervene by diplomacy or by force when human rights are being contravened. The International Convention on Human Rights and the European Convention on Human Rights set out the rights that should be afforded to any individual by virtue of being human. These rights are protected in law and articulated in Britain through the Human Rights Act (1998) (see Figure 1.1).

The Human Rights Act (1998) sets out 16 basic rights that all people in Britain should enjoy.

1 The right to life (Article 2)
2 Prohibition of torture (Article 3)
3 Prohibition of slavery and forced labour (Article 4)
4 Right to liberty and security (Article 5)
5 Right to a fair trial (Article 6)
6 No punishment without law (Article 7)
7 Right to respect for private and family life (Article 8)
8 Freedom of thought, conscience and religion (Article 9)
9 Freedom of expression (Article 10)
10 Right to freedom of assembly and association (Article 11)
11 The right to marry (Article 12)
12 Prohibition of discrimination (Article 14)
13 Protection of property (Article 1 of Protocol 1)
14 Right to education (Article 2 of Protocol 1)
15 Right to free elections (Article 3 of Protocol 1)
16 Abolition of the death penalty (Article 1 of Protocol 6).

Figure 1.1 The Human Rights Act (1998)

When these rights are violated, a citizen has the right to challenge this violation and, where relevant, seek appropriate action or compensation.

A number of these rights are more relevant to the health and care context than others. Since the Human Rights Act (1998) became operational in

2001 a number of cases have been brought to court. For example, the prohibition of torture has been used to bring cases against local authorities who failed to protect children from abuse. The right to liberty is relevant to the detention of individuals under the Mental Health Act (1983). Freedom from discrimination has been used by the Disability Rights Commission fighting the case for equality of opportunity and treatment for disabled people (Department of Health, 2005a). Challenges under the Human Rights Act (1998) are not as common as was first feared when the Act was introduced. However, the care practitioner needs to be aware of the articles that are enshrined in British law.

Legal rights

Legal rights are those rights that are enshrined in law and that society seeks to uphold by promise and through the justice system when these rights are challenged. For example, there is a legal right to equal pay for the same job.

Moral rights

Moral rights are rights that are associated with the manner in which people are treated. These rights may be identified through explicit public declarations of values and behaviours such as in professional codes, or they may be culturally assumed through the adoption of belief and value systems such as the adoption of particular religious doctrines. These rights are much harder to protect as they are often not clearly defined and are not always shared by everyone.

Negative rights or liberty rights

Negative or liberty rights do not require an individual to make a claim, nor to require another to provide something or do something. A negative right relates to the freedom to do something without interference. For example, the freedom of speech and the right to practise one's preferred religion (or the right not to practise a religion).

LIMITATIONS ON RIGHTS

It is important to recognise that, although rights are an important consideration in our culture, rights are rarely absolute and rights can be curtailed. If, in exercising my right to freedom of speech, I override other rights by making sexist or racist remarks, I can have my right to freedom of speech legally curtailed or infringed. That infringement only applies to those remarks that are in breach of anti-discriminatory laws and does not apply to my freedom of speech generally. This is a justified infringement of my rights. If, however, my rights are 'violated', this is an unjustified infringement of my rights. For example, if I decide that I do not want to take part in a research project, but you decide that you can give me the trial treatment without me realising and therefore go ahead with this, my rights to refuse treatment and my right of informed consent will have been violated. The important point to note here is that at times, usually in extreme circumstances, rights will need to be infringed. However, when rights are being infringed in any way it is important that that infringement can be justified.

Question

Can you think of any examples of justified infringements of rights in a care context? How would you justify them?

RIGHTS IN CARE

The rights of users in care services are more specific than those labelled human rights or even citizen rights. User rights are those entitlements that apply specifically to users of a care service. They are clearly articulated in patients' charters and documents outlining the rights for specific groups like, for example, its rights to care and treatment (in mental health) (Rethink; www.rethink.org), the duties and responsibilities of care workers in their codes of practice (see the GSCC *Code of Practice* (GSCC, 2002)), in declarations from service providers such as, for example, *The Patient's Charter* (DoH, 1997), and in the publication of standards of service and legislation.

Rights, needs and wants

In relation to care provision it is important to distinguish between 'rights', 'needs' and 'wants'. Public expectations are often confused in terms of what they would like and what they are entitled to. Wants are often expressed in terms of rights as it appears that these claims will have more legitimacy. It is important for the care worker to be able to differentiate between reasonable and justified claims and wants, and to be able to articulate differences between these two things.

A *need* is a requirement. It is something where it can be demonstrated that the individual will suffer a significant harm if they are denied it (Doyal and Gough, 1991). A *want* is something that an individual would like, and which might even be desirable to provide, if the resources are available.

However, a want is neither an entitlement nor a requirement so, therefore, it should not be provided over the entitlements or needs of others.

As discussed earlier in the chapter, a right is something to which one is entitled. This may apply universally or be restricted to a specific group.In care provision, entitlements to care are often justified in terms of the level of need. The greater the need, the greater the entitlement to the provision. Therefore, those with more severe difficulties should be able to make a stronger claim to have their needs met. While it is not always that simple, because these claims will be restricted by available resources, needs assessment will provide a 'rule of thumb' for helping workers to differentiate between competing claims.

Writing activity

Make a list of the rights that you think recipients of care services should be entitled to and identify why you think these rights should be upheld. Your list might include some of those identified in the rest of this chapter.

The right to be treated with respect and dignity

This principle was articulated in the 1994 Declaration on the Promotion of Patient Rights in Europe and is the basis for national laws and charters on user and patient rights. Dignity and respect are key concepts within professional codes of practice and within the NHS Plan (DoH, 2000). It is based on the belief that illness and vulnerability are not reasons to be treated less well than other people.

Definitions of respect and dignity

Even though an individual may find themselves in a vulnerable or dependent situation they are entitled to the same level of dignity, respect and protection that can be expected by anyone in that society. This right is justified on grounds of our shared humanity. The fact that we are all human means that we share a common set of values and, therefore, that no one is entitled to more, or less, dignity and respect than others.

Dignity and respect, like many commonly used terms in care, do not have a simple definition, but they can be broadly defined as being 'worthy of self-esteem' and having the 'esteem of others'. Seedhouse and Gallagher (2002) link dignity and respect to our capabilities and the opportunity to exercise those capabilities effectively. This definition helps us understand the concepts – think about how you feel when your dignity is infringed, or when your capabilities are compromised or thwarted by another. Lack of respect and dignity may leave us feeling devalued, worthless, frustrated and angry because it is a fundamental assault on the individual as a human It could be argued that care workers are privileged. By virtue of the nature of their work they are invited to be involved in intimate aspects of others' lives. They may be engaged in physical care or be privy to personal affairs such as financial information, family relationships, knowledge of personal needs and so on. This means that people in receipt of care, by necessity, have less opportunity to maintain their privacy than others. However, this detailed knowledge of others could also be the reason why dignity, privacy and respect are infringed. Over-familiarity, thinking that you know better than the person themselves about what is good for them, and the unin-vited sharing of information with others are all examples of how care workers can infringe the rights and dignity of those in their care, even though this is often done with the best intentions of the care worker. Care that respects dignity must therefore be sensitive to the feelings and needs and rights of others in order that they can enjoy, as near as possible, the same level of respect and privacy as those not in receipt of care. Care workers must therefore develop good communication skills so that they can detect and interpret others' feelings, listen attentively to their needs and to communicate necessary information effectively in a manner that does not patronise or dictate.

Discussion activity

It is important to reflect on your own approach to the care of others. Tick the words in the lists below that best reflect your beliefs about care and discuss this with a colleague.

Support	Help
Educate	Inform
Independence	Protect
Equality	Power
Risk	Persuade
Partnership	Responsibility
Listen	Consult

A paternalistic approach to care

All of the words in the two lists above reflect appropriate behaviours in care. However, different approaches to care need to be used selectively. If you ticked more words in the second list you may have a more

protective or 'paternalistic' approach to care. When people feel particularly vulnerable a paternalistic approach to care can be the most
appropriate because it relieves the stress and responsibility of decision-making. However, it is not normally desirable to sustain this
approach to care. In a paternalistic relationship the power resides
with the care giver. This means that it creates a dependent relationship
in which the recipient relies heavily on the care giver. The danger of this
approach to care is that it does not create an environment in which the
recipient can develop, take risks or become independent. In addition, it
is likely that in such a relationship the views of the carer are going to be
dominant and may even conflict with those of the service user. If the
care giver then persuades the recipient into a particular unwanted
course of action they have not respected the individual's dignity. A
paternalistic approach might therefore be selected at times when an
individual requires more than average support. However, such an
approach should be administered with great care to ensure that the
support and protection offered by this approach to care do not inadvertently become unnecessarily controlling and that, as far as possible,
the approach maintains the right of service users to be treated with
respect and dignity.

A care facilitator

If your approach in the activity above reflected words mainly in the first
list, you may see yourself primarily as someone who facilitates care, i.e.,
someone who supports others to lead their own lives. You are adopting an
approach that recognises the dignity, individuality and autonomy of the
recipient. While this approach to care encourages independence and
personal development, there is a danger that this may fail to protect
the vulnerable person adequately. It may also bring the care worker
into conflict with the user, who may be reluctant to take responsibility
and make choices. Users may make poor choices or be ill-informed, which
could leave the care worker feeling frustrated or angry. In this approach to
care the role of the care giver is to promote the right of individuals to
make choices, to provide appropriate information to enable those choices
to be made and, where possible, to support the opportunity to put these
choices into action. The obligation that comes with facilitating decision-
making is to have the courage to allow people to carry their decision-
making through, even though this may be accompanied by risks.

People do not choose to be in poverty, or ill or elderly. These are states in
which anyone of us can find ourselves, at any time and for varying periods
of our lives. At such times our vulnerability should not provide an excuse
for others to treat us less well than other members of society. In fact, it
could be argued that vulnerability should require that greater efforts are

made by others to uphold our dignity because the need is greater. It is clear that a 'one size fits all' approach to care is inappropriate and that the care worker must be guided by the needs of the recipient. However dignity and respect must be maintained no matter which approach is adopted.

The right to be treated fairly

This right supports the notion that I should not be treated differently from others for irrelevant reasons. In relation to care this can be interpreted as the right to access the same services and provision as others in a similar situation to myself. Being treated fairly does not always mean that I should have exactly the same things as other people. The principle of fairness suggests that, where a need is identified, I am treated no less favourably than those who have a similar need, irrespective of my personal attributes. This right is easy to explain in terms of service provision, but it is equally true of hands-on one-to-one care. The personal care that is received should be of the same standard as that received by others in terms of the quality and competence of the care provided, the time allocated for that care delivery and the attitude with which the care is delivered. It may be preferable to provide care to someone who is grateful or who is interesting, who is in a particular age group or for whom one has a personal affinity. However, these are irrelevant grounds for distinguishing between people. All people are entitled to the same fair level of care provision irrespective of their attributes.

Right to confidentiality

We have the right to have information about us kept confidential, or to know on what basis information will be shared with others. This subject will be addressed in depth in Chapter 4. Therefore, we will only make the point here that confidentiality is, in most cases, a right as long as it does not impinge on the rights or protection of others.

The right to ordinary life opportunities

Being in receipt of care is not an excuse for settling for a second-rate life. The role of welfare provision is to try to ensure service users/patients have access to the same kind of opportunities enjoyed by other members of that community. Therefore, people should have the opportunity to access treatments that support illness, or to transport such as wheelchairs if mobility is compromised, or to social networks or access to activities that most people enjoy. The right of the recipient of care is to have access to supportive facilities that enable them to avail themselves of the opportunities that others take for granted.

The right to competent care provision from service providers

This right means that the people providing care will be more than just 'nice people'. It means that a user has the right to receive care from someone who has received the appropriate level of training to provide the care that the user needs. In addition, the practitioner will recognise when they have reached their limitations and will know how to access appropriate help or support. However, competent care is not just about technical ability. Care practitioners, therefore, have a duty to ensure that their skills are up to date and appropriate for the care they are providing. This right has been endorsed in health and care by the growth of evidence-based care. It is no longer acceptable to continue a practice and justify it on grounds that 'we have always done it that way'. There is now a huge quantity of easily accessible evidence and practitioners have a duty to try to keep informed about changes in their own field of practice. Equally, employers have an obligation to ensure that opportunities for training and updating are made available to practitioners. Care implies an element of compassion and therefore competent care will not involve treating service users as machines. It will involve sensitivity, respect for needs and the ways in which the recipient would like their needs to be met.

The right to independent advocacy when requested

At times individuals may not be able to articulate their own needs effectively. In such cases they may need support from someone who can speak on their behalf. Care workers may not be the best people to undertake this role. They may be constrained by professional requirements and obligations to an employer or by a particular point of view. They may also be too closely involved or swayed by their own knowledge and interpretation of the individual's needs and hence be unable to reflect those needs accurately. Where users are unable to articulate their own needs they must have the right to access someone who will speak on their behalf.

To be accepted for what one is

This right can be seen to embrace the important concepts of equality and anti-discriminatory practice. These rights have been enshrined in law for longer than most other aspects of the Human Rights Act and they are fundamental to protecting the dignity of minority groups and vulnerable individuals. As such, they warrant some in-depth discussion later in this chapter.

CELEBRATING DIFFERENCE

One of the most prized aspects of human beings is their individuality. No two people are the same. Even identical twins, who share the same genetic code, will display differences in a number of ways. Each one of us wants to be recognised by our own individual identity and personality and to be seen as an independent and worthwhile person in our own right. We seek to illustrate this in the values we adopt, in the activities we engage in and the way we dress (how uncomfortable is it when someone else is wearing the same clothes as you?). The point is that we go to great lengths to make sure that we are different from those around us. At this level, when we think about ourselves, difference is good.

Writing activity

Think about your friends. Try to identify the ways in which they are different and what you value about their different attributes.

Hopefully, your friends are not all the same and you value a whole range of attributes in others, relating to your friends in different ways and for different purposes. For example, you may have one friend who is your confidant, who provides sound advice, or who is just a good listener. However, when you want a friend for a light fun evening out you may choose a different friend. These differences do not make either friend less valuable than the other; it is just recognition of difference. These differences are the things that make us interesting. Difference is therefore something to be celebrated.

Imaginative exercise

Imagine a time when it becomes common practice to treat all people with blond hair with contempt, either by ignoring them or treating them less well than those with hair of any other colour. This treatment is widely accepted by the rest of society.
1. Could this behaviour be rationalised?
2. Should I expect everyone with blond hair to dye it brown in order that they would not be discriminated against?

Given that blond hair for many people is a matter of genetic lottery, it would seem to be laughable to suggest that one's worth could be based on such flimsy grounds. However, this is exactly what we do when we discriminate against those who have a disability, a different race, a particular sexuality or other less tangible characteristics. Individuals may be victimised, ignored or expected to change into something that accords with our beliefs and expectations. The thing that makes humans so interesting and so valuable is their difference. We should celebrate it, not penalise people for it.

When a difference is something we have not encountered before or is something we do not understand, we may feel threatened. Rather than celebrating the difference and trying to see the value of it, we may react negatively. Education in relation to equality and anti-discriminatory practice is designed to help us better understand difference and our reactions to difference, and help us to respect others and value them for what they are.

Equality and anti-discriminatory practice are important considerations in a free and tolerant society that respects and prizes individuality. Likewise, in care practice that supports the notion of the value of the individual, equality and anti-discriminatory practice are important concepts. Both concepts suggest the notion of fairness and justice.

There are numerous policies and legislation in respect of equality and anti-discriminatory practice. Some of the key Acts are the Human Rights Act (1998), the Disability Discrimination Act (2005), the Race Relations Act (2000) and the Equality and Human Rights Act (2006). However, despite this legislation, it remains a fact that inequality and discrimination still persist in health and social care, and policy will only go some of the way to challenge discrimination. What is crucially important is how that policy is implemented and embedded within day-to-day interactions between practitioners and those in their care.

UNDERSTANDING EQUALITY, PREJUDICE AND DISCRIMINATION

Much of the literature on discrimination and inequality focuses particularly on vulnerable groups like, for example, older people, those with disabilities, women, those of different race, people with mental health problems or those of different sexual orientation. It is, of course, important to focus on the specific difficulties faced by individuals in these groups. However, it should not be forgotten that anyone can be discriminated against at any time and the discrimination may have no discernible basis or may be based on a dislike or something equally insubstantial. In addressing issues of equality and discrimination it is important to understand what is meant by the terms used.

Equality

Equality does not mean treating everyone the same. Just as people are different, so their needs are different. What is important is that the same principles of fairness are used to establish their need and subsequent treatment. Therefore, equality implies that they should be treated fairly.

Applying the principle of equality in practice means that all people in similar situations should be treated similarly. Therefore, all people with a particular type of breast cancer should be offered the same options for treatment. They may not all choose to access the same treatment because their decision will be based on a range of different considerations. However, equality requires that the same opportunities exist for everyone. It is unrealistic to suggest that everyone will be treated exactly the same and situational differences and the dynamics of human interaction make this unlikely, if not impossible. However, there should be no significant differences in treatment unless that difference can be appropriately and convincingly justified.

Reflection

Try to think of examples from your own experience of care of people being treated differently even though they had similarities in their needs. Can you suggest reasons for differences in the treatment of individuals and are these reasons persuasive?

You may be looking after two individuals who have had to leave their homes for full-time care in a care home. One of the individuals has made the choice voluntarily and is happy to be there. One has had to reluctantly admit that she can no longer cope and sees the care home as her only option. While it would be very important to help both women settle in well, you may find that you need to adopt very different strategies to do this. Treating people differently may be entirely justifiable as long as the principle of fairness is understood and applied, as a check, and that any material difference can be appropriately explained.

Failure to respect another's right to equality puts them at a disadvantage. It is recognised that unequal treatment, at times, arises from naivety or the ineffectiveness of the practitioner, and in situations where no malice is intended, but this is still unacceptable practice. It is not difficult to see how the needs of a demanding person can take precedence over the needs of someone who sits and waits patiently for their care. However, even though such inequality is non-intentional, it should be guarded against.

Prejudice

Inequality is much more unacceptable when it takes the form of prejudice and/or discrimination. Prejudice is an attitude or belief based on a faulty and inflexible generalisation (Allport, 1954). Discrimination can be defined as unequal and unfair treatment that is usually based on prejudice. Discrimination and prejudice are very loaded words and are usually associated with negative connotations, but discrimination and prejudice can be positive or favourable in nature. That is, we can hold a particular prejudice that causes us to positively discriminate in favour of someone. For example, we can hold a belief that someone who speaks with a southern BBC English accent will be a better candidate for a job than someone who has a strong regional accent, irrespective of their other skills. This is unfair positive prejudice and is the result of drawing inappropriate conclusions from irrelevant evidence. However, there are examples of positive discrimination that help us to combat prejudice. For example, the Disability Discrimination Act (2005) requires organisations to try to recruit individuals with disabilities because, as a group, it is known that they experience significant prejudice and unfair discrimination on irrelevant grounds that have nothing to do with the ability to do the job.

Writing activity

Make a note of other examples of effective and welcome positive prejudice.

Normally, however, when we talk about prejudice we are thinking of negative examples of applying faulty and negative generalisations. An example might be the statement 'people are unemployed because they are lazy'. Although this assertion may apply to a small minority, there is substantial evidence to the contrary. It is more widely accepted and demonstrated in research that there is a multitude of complex reasons why someone is unemployed. Prejudice can be directed at a group as a whole, or an individual because they are a member of a group. This is justified by the person holding the prejudice by ascribing particular stereotypical attributes and behaviours to the individual or group who are the focus of the prejudice, as a means of attempting to explain why the prejudice is held. Stereotypical views such as 'women are emotional and illogical' or 'men are hard and logical' are widely held and believed, even in the face of evidence to the contrary.

How does prejudice manifest itself?

According to Allport (1954), a prejudice may involve a number of processes.

- **Cognitive** – you develop a false belief that one person or group is better or superior to another (this belief may develop at a conscious or at an unconscious level – you may, for example, have acquired it from your parents or friends).
- **Emotional** – this belief provokes an emotional response, a feeling towards a particular individual or group, that may be dislike or dismissal.
- **Discriminatory action** – this feeling may then be manifested in a number of ways, for example, ignoring the person, saying unpleasant things about them to others, deliberately humiliating them, or taking some other form of unfair action against them.

Prejudices can be held without resorting to discrimination and discrimination can occur without prejudice. However, there is frequently a very close and causal link between the two.

Examining prejudice makes individuals feel uncomfortable and most of us would prefer to believe that we do not hold any prejudices. However, it is true to say that we all hold some prejudices. What is important is that we accept that we will always hold some, we learn to recognise them and we try to eliminate them but, where we cannot, we develop strategies so that they do not lead us into engaging in discriminatory behaviours. Thompson (2006) reminds us that prejudice and subsequent discrimination are rarely confined to the beliefs and actions of an individual but are the result of a combination of influences.

- **Personal beliefs** – those beliefs and values held and acted upon by an individual.
- **Cultural beliefs** – those values held in the social environment that an individual inhabits that strongly influence the individual. For example, a few years ago, following the Stephen Lawrence enquiry the police service was accused of being 'institutionally racist'.
- **Social and structural beliefs** – these reflect the established social order and are the influence of beliefs, values and divisions in our wider society. There are a number of examples of discriminatory practice of this nature including the fact that it is only very recently (2006) that the law recognised same-sex partnerships.

The evidence that inequality and discrimination in health and care services persist is overwhelming.

- The NHS continues to be the service about which the Commission for Racial Equality receives most complaints (CRE, 2005).
- The formal investigation into *Equal treatment: closing the gap*, by the Disabilities Rights Commission (2006), demonstrates that people with disabilities die earlier than able-bodied people and experience more illness but face greater barriers than able-bodied people in securing the care services that they need (DRC, 2006).
- People over 65 experience significant discrimination in health and care services (Help the Aged, 2007).

This evidence of ongoing prejudice and discrimination suggests that care workers are inadequately prepared to work in a non-judgemental and anti-discriminatory manner.

Why do discrimination and prejudice continue to exist in care?

All codes of practice in the fields of health and social care emphasise the need to engage in non-judgemental and anti-discriminatory practice. However, discrimination still persists. There are a number of reasons why this could be so.

- Individuals have a poor or limited understanding of prejudice and anti-discriminatory practice.
- Wherever small groups of workers work in teams there is a tendency to develop particular sets of practices and behaviours. Charles Handy (1997) has likened this to tribes who hold sets of specific and often exclusive tribal behaviours. Prejudices, because they can be unconsciously held, can thrive in these environments and might not be recognised by those who belong to that group. New staff to an area may initially be aware of prejudicial practices but, as they become part of the everyday experience (as long as the practices are not extreme), the new staff member may quickly adapt to the behaviours themselves in an effort to belong to the existing group, and so the behaviours are perpetuated.
- There are organisational policies or constraints which support discriminatory practice.
- The power imbalance between the carer and the cared for supports an environment in which the individual in receipt of care will always be at risk of anti-discriminatory behaviour.
- Likes and dislikes of individuals or groups can result in discrimination.
- Care practitioners may believe that individuals who are different should, as far as possible, conform to the majority or less different position.

ENGAGING IN ANTI-DISCRIMINATORY PRACTICE

Treating service users fairly is one of the core duties of a care practitioner. Unfair treatment increases vulnerability and causes disadvantage. There are a number of principles that emerge from literature regarding how inequality and discrimination can be tackled in practice. Twelvetrees (2002) suggests ways of tackling inequality by changing our approach, by:

- celebrating diversity – reframing difference so that sharing different views and accepting different choices are positive activities that enhance our knowledge and experience;
- challenging oppression – when we see oppression from others we should question and challenge it, or refuse to be part of it;
- empowering the oppressed – power or perceived power is often exercised by those who engage in discrimination so, if we can help to empower those who are seen as vulnerable, we can help break the cycle of discrimination.

Gilchrist (1992) suggests a number of steps that must be taken to ensure anti-discriminatory practice can become embedded. These include:

- recognise prejudice and the discriminatory practices that this leads to;
- value diversity;
- understand a need to find ways to empower others;
- combat discrimination and encourage others to combat discrimination;
- reflect on the organisation and the policies, procedures, practices and facilities which might support discriminatory practices.

How can these principles be applied to a care environment?

Celebrate diversity

Even if you work with one service user group, think about the things that make each individual different. Even when you do not particularly like someone it is usually possible to find a redeeming feature or some attribute that you admire, so focus on the positive not the negative.

Challenge oppression

When people talk in denigratory ways about others we should question it and refuse to condone racist or sexist jokes that reinforce stereotypes and prejudice. Ask questions about why certain practices are done as this may bring hitherto unrecognised issues into the open. There is no need to be directly confrontational; merely not engaging in the practice or questioning something stops the reinforcement of it.

Empowering the oppressed

In recent years the introduction of advocacy schemes and user and carer involvement initiatives go some way to empowering others. However, empowerment need not be at this formal level but can be as simple as establishing a relationship of equality and respect with the individual in your care and taking time to listen to and, where possible, action their views and needs.

Recognising prejudice

It is essential to reflect on your own possible prejudices. We cannot begin to combat something if we do not acknowledge that it exists. Ask yourself questions such as: 'what prejudices do I hold?', 'where do they come from and why?' Challenge your prejudices. Examine your care practice. Did you spend more time or better quality time with one client rather than another client? Why was this? Is there any evidence that it was based on prejudice? What strategies could you use to overcome your prejudices?

> **Reflection**
>
> Reflect on the organisation and context in which you deliver care. Does the organisation reinforce discrimination or support anti-discriminatory practice?

These are examples of how you can begin to think about anti-discriminatory practice and embed the principles of this in your own practice.

- Are there any policies or practices that discriminate against individuals on the basis of age?
- Do you have any practices that favour opportunities for one service user over another?
- Are there any areas that are inaccessible to some service users because of their disabilities?
- Do you provide interpretation for those whose first language is not English?

- Do you hold service user meetings at a time or venue where it is difficult for users to attend?
- Do you have a philosophy in the organisation that promotes empowerment?

Case study

Mrs Kowalski is a Jewish lady of Polish origin who has just started coming to the day centre in which you work. When you come on duty you are told that she is introverted and difficult. She has not eaten or drunk anything that has been given to her, she refuses to join in the activities that are put on and seems reluctant to answer questions. She has been incontinent twice and staff are considering whether she is a suitable candidate for this service, which would be better going to someone else who would appreciate it. You notice that staff are avoiding contact with her. This is the first time that Mrs Kowalski has been in a care environment. She does not speak English well and has difficulty hearing people because of her deteriorating hearing. She has been an orthodox Jew all her life and only eats kosher food.

1. Which of Mrs Kowalski's rights are not being met?

2. What could you do in order to improve her experience of care?

A RIGHTS-BASED APPROACH TO CARE

It may have become obvious that a rights-focused approach to care is aimed at protecting and furthering the independence of and opportunities for all individuals, and that it is a particularly useful tool for vulnerable people to use to challenge unfair treatment, inequality and discrimination. However, rights cannot be easily separated from responsibilities. In the discussion about rights far less attention has been paid to the corresponding responsibilities that go hand-in-hand with many rights. It needs to be recognised that if I am to be in receipt of rights then it must be on the basis that someone has agreed to provide that right and will go on and action that agreement. If they fail in this duty, in relation to an explicit right, there is a case to answer. However, I, as the recipient of rights, might also have responsibilities. If I want to have the right to have my individual needs met I must accept the responsibility that I must try to articulate effectively what those needs are; it is unreasonable to expect another to guess what those specific needs might be. I may also be responsible for working in partnership with the care provider to ensure that the rights can be met.

What happens when rights conflict?

Earlier in the chapter it was stated that, although I have rights, these are not absolute and can be negotiated, curtailed or infringed. Rights do conflict and it is beholden on care workers to recognise these conflicts and, where possible, resolve them. Good communication is essential. Do you know what the service user's expectations are? Does the service user know to what they are entitled? Where it is impossible to meet conflicting rights, can you negotiate with the service user to identify which rights are more important to them, or explain why one right needs to take precedence over another? Rights conflicts may never be resolved to everyone's satisfaction but good communication, that is open and honest about what can and cannot be achieved, and why, will go a long way to helping individuals cope with the feeling of powerlessness that is so often experienced when one feels one's rights have not been respected.

At times the rights of one person will conflict with another's. Resolution can be difficult and usually involves a decision about which rights need to take precedence. This decision may be arbitrary or unfairly administered. At times rights issues are resolved through the resort to law such as, for example, the right to an assisted death that was unsuccessfully challenged by Dianne Pretty, who had motor neurone disease. Where different people can demonstrate an equal claim to have their rights upheld, but these claims conflict, there may be no way of reaching a resolution in a rights-based approach to care. However, the rights-based approach to care works well for individuals and groups who are protecting themselves against discrimination and unfair treatment. This approach is based on the idea of a contract and is only really effective if all parties keep their side of the contract. Finally, it is important to realise that the concept of rights is one that is strongly held in Western, democratic societies but is not a concept that translates effectively to all cultures.

CONCLUSION

A rights-based approach to care is based upon the core values of care and rights are claimed against those core values. Rights claims are often made when individuals feel that their rights are not being met or that they are being treated unfairly, and when they have exhausted all other avenues and there are no other options for their needs to be heard. The problem is that asserting rights and claims can be very confrontational and divisive. It can be argued that a rights-based society can lead to a society in which individuals selfishly care more about the fulfilment of their individual rights than they do about the state of society as a whole, or about individuals who are in a worse situation than themselves. An alternative approach is for society to strive to identify the rights and respect that all citizens should enjoy and ensure that this respect and these rights are afforded to all, without an individual having to fight for them. However, this discussion is beyond the scope of this chapter.

SUMMARY OF KEY POINTS
- Rights are an important feature of care in Western societies.
- There are many different kinds of rights.
- Rights are often resorted to when individuals feel they are not receiving that to which they are entitled.
- Rights provide a vehicle for people to articulate their needs.
- Discriminatory practices still occur in care practice.
- Practitioners need to reflect on their practice and develop strategies to eliminate discrimination.

FURTHER READING

Bateman, N. (2006) *Practising welfare rights* (Social Work Skills series). London: Routledge

Disability Rights website: **www.direct.gov.uk/en/DisabledPeople/ RightsAndObligations/Disability Rights/index.htm**

Discrimination website: **www.direct.gov.uk**

Equality and Human Rights Commission website: **www.equalityhuman-rights.com/pages/eocdrccre.aspx**

Roy, L. (2001) *Understanding the Human Rights Act: a toolkit for the health service*. Abingdon: Radcliffe Medical

Chapter 2

Respect and Dignity

Key themes

In this chapter you will:

- define respect and dignity and consider what it means to be respectful and have respect for others;

- explore the concepts of respect, dignity and privacy in relation to practice;

- be introduced to a moral justification for a duty of respect for persons and consider the notion of personhood;

- examine duties and rules arising from respect for persons and their implications for practice;

- reflect on care strategies that promote respect and dignity.

INTRODUCTION

People generally value their independence and the opportunity to maintain control over their own lives. Recognition of your humanity through respect for you as a person is fundamental to maintaining your dignity and to your feelings of self-esteem and self-worth. These notions of respect and dignity have attracted considerable attention in recent years, both in theory and in practice. They are at the forefront of current government policy and have been reflected in a range of government reports, with claims of increasing opportunities for individual choice and involvement in decision-making about health and care services (Department of Health (DoH), 2005a, 2006). The value of respect and dignity has been specifically highlighted in relation to groups of service users who may be particularly vulnerable to feelings of loss of self-worth and at risk of being treated differently or with disrespect, including older people, those with learning disabilities or those with mental health problems.

For example, the National Service Framework (NSF) for Older People (DoH, 2001a) was triggered by concerns about widespread infringement of dignity and unfair discrimination in older people's access to care. *Valuing people: a new strategy for learning disability for the 21st century* (DoH, 2001b) emphasises the importance of person-centred approaches in working with people with learning disabilities and their carers, and respect is also at the heart of the Best Practice Guidance *Capabilities for inclusive practice in mental health* (DoH, 2007). However, the values of respect for persons and dignity are not exclusive to particular service user groups. They are relevant to whoever you will meet in your practice, including staff and other carers, and in your everyday life.

The expectation that you will practise with respect for people and for their autonomy and dignity is also reinforced by a number, if not all, of the competencies within the National Occupational Standards for Health and Social Care and these concepts underpin the rights of individuals as defined by Skills for Care (Skills for Care, 2005) (see Figure 2.1) as well as being emphasised in the *Essence of Care* Benchmark for 'Privacy and Dignity' (DoH, 2003a).

The National Occupational Standards for Health and Social Care 2005 identify that individuals and key people have the right to:

- be respected;
- be treated equally and not be discriminated against;
- be treated as an individual;
- be treated in a dignified way;
- privacy;
- be protected from danger and harm;
- be cared for in the way that meets their needs, takes account of their choices and also protects them;
- access information about themselves;
- communicate using their preferred methods of communication and language.

See, for example, Skills for Health Competence HSC3112: 'Support individuals to identify and promote their own health and social well being' at **www.skillsfor-health.org.uk/tools/viewcomp.php?id=1360** (accessed 16 July 2007).

Figure 2.1 Definition of rights taken from key words and concepts in the National Occupational Standards for Health and Social Care 2005

The concepts of respect, autonomy and preserving dignity are also funda-mental to many codes of practice and professional conduct for health and care practitioners including, for example, the *Code of Practice for Social*

Care Workers (General Social Care Council, 2002), *The NMC Code of Professional Conduct: standards for conduct, performance and ethics*, which is currently under consultation (Nursing and Midwifery Council, 2004) and the *College of Occupational Therapists Code of Ethics and Professional Conduct* (College of Occupational Therapists, 2005). However, these concepts are more complex in their meaning and their application than any of these rules for practice alone can convey.

The concept of dignity in itself can be hard to define but what is clear is that people recognise when they have not been treated with dignity and respect (Healthcare Commission, 2007; SCIE, 2006). Dignity is most closely associated with the notions of respect (of self and others), respect for persons and having respect for a person's autonomy, i.e. the capacity to be one's own person and make choices and decisions about how their lives should go. Harris (1985, p.193) adds 'having concern for the welfare of others' as another essential component of respect for persons. This is normally mutually compatible with respect for autonomy, although many moral dilemmas in health and social care practice arise when these two come into conflict, as you will see later in this chapter and in Chapter 5 when we talk about risk and acting in a person's best interests.

Being worthy of respect and the value placed on dignity are based in our shared humanity and the intrinsic value attributed to every human being. One important implication of respect for persons and human dignity is that every person should be acknowledged as an inherently valuable member of the community and as a unique individual entitled to the same level of respect as any other. Respect for persons and human dignity should have no boundaries and go beyond any social order such that they cannot be legitimately violated by society. In this way, respect for persons and dignity are the basis for human rights and are fundamental to our feelings of self-esteem and self-worth.

This chapter aims to develop your deeper understanding of the values of respect for persons and dignity and Chapter 3 focuses on respect for autonomy. Both chapters aim to help you to reflect on care strategies that promote respect, dignity and autonomy in order to inform and improve your practice.

WHAT DO WE MEAN WHEN WE USE THE TERMS 'RESPECT' AND 'RESPECT FOR PERSONS'?

Thinking about respect as a value

Respect is important to daily life, although you may feel that this has too often been equated with simply respecting the authority of, for example, people in power, the law or religion. The word 'respect' is becoming more commonplace in everyday language, both in the general public domain (for example, respecting nature and the environment, respect for human life in debates about abortion, respecting cultural difference and diversity) and in political debate like, for example, the *Respect Action Plan* published in 2006 by the Labour government, which set out to build a modern culture of respect aimed at tackling anti-social behaviour and improving community cohesion (see Figure 2.2 – The 'Respect drive').

This is a cross-government strategy to tackle bad behaviour and nurture good – and so help create the modern culture of respect.

'It is about central government, local agencies, local communities and ultimately every citizen working together to build a society in which we can respect one another – where anti-social behaviour is rare and tackled effectively, and communities can live in peace together.

It's not about going back to the past or returning to the days of 'knowing your place'. It's about nurturing and, where needed, enforcing a modern culture of respect, which the majority of people want.

It's about showing tolerance, acceptance and common decency towards the people around us – our family, friends and peers, people who are older or younger than us, people from different walks of life or who follow different cultures or religions. It's about being considerate of the consequences of our behaviour for others.

For most of us this is automatic and ingrained in the habits of our everyday lives. But when respect for self, others and the community breaks down, anti-social behaviour takes hold.

Making offensive and threatening remarks, dumping litter and urinating in the street are clearly inconsiderate or disrespectful by any definition.

Respect or the lack of it does more than affect us as individuals. Understanding and adopting a code of behaviour is what makes society work as a whole and is why the government is so committed to working with the public to promote a new culture of respect.

Taken from the government's 'Respect' website at **www.respect.gov. uk/article.aspx?id=9054** (accessed 16 May 2007)

Figure 2.2 The 'Respect drive'

Aside from government action, respect for self and others can be seen as a fundamental element of living together in a society. However, there are many ways to think about and use the term 'respect' and it may have different meanings to different people and according to the context in which it is used, such as, 'respect me for who I am' or 'respect my authority'. Both of these demand acknowledgment, recognition and consideration by others although the reason for giving (or owing) such respect is different.

Reflection

Have you ever experienced a time when you felt that you were not respected or felt undervalued? This may have been, for example, in a family or personal relationship, in an interaction with someone you know or with a stranger, or in a work environment.

1. Describe this significant incident. Where were you? Who was involved? Were there any specific circumstances?

2. Then think about and write down:
   a. How did this make you feel?
   b. Why did you feel this way?
   c. What did you do?

You may have identified a number of feelings like, for example, anger, upset, sadness, disbelief, concern, being belittled. It may have been harder to identify exactly why you felt this way; you may have said, 'It just wasn't "fair" or "right"'. However, it's important as a reflective practitioner that you keep asking yourself why you believe something is right or wrong or should or should not be the way it is. You may have said that it was disrespectful of you as an individual. This idea of respect and respect for persons needs further exploration.

Defining respect

There are many different ways to define and think about respect. The term 'respect' can refer simply to a behaviour that avoids violating or interfering with a boundary or rule; for example, a driver respecting a speed limit or a smoker refraining from smoking in public places in respect of the ban imposed by changes in legislation. Respect can also involve an attitude or feeling, as when we speak of having respect for another person. As practitioners in health and care you will have to respect boundaries or rules such as, for example, the law associated with consent to treatment, policies, competencies for practice and the rules outlined in codes of conduct. However, what we are most concerned about here are the values and attitudes associated with 'respect for persons' and their influence on your behaviours and practice.

Writing activity

1. Think about and write down your definition of 'respect'.

2. If you find this difficult, do a 'spider diagram' showing different words, phrases and ideas that come to mind when you think about 'respect' (redraw the diagram in the centre of an A4 piece of paper as you may well identify many more words and ideas than indicated by the six arrows below).

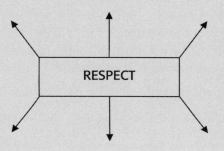

3. Look up 'respect' in a dictionary and add the definition to your 'mind map' (but remember a dictionary definition will only start to identify its meaning).

4. Now talk to some relatives, friends and/or colleagues about their understanding of the term 'respect'.

5. Try rewriting your definition now.

Respect in this context can be simply defined as the recognition of the unconditional value of patients, service users, clients and carers as persons. This requires both a belief that persons should be valued and that your actions should reflect such a belief (Beach *et al.*, 2007). Respect seen in this way necessarily involves respecting autonomy but this alone is not a sufficient understanding of respect for persons in care relationships. Therefore, respect can mean:

- a symbolic recognition of status or social position;
- paying heed to or giving proper attention to the 'object' of respect;
- acknowledgement of the value, worth and importance of something or someone.

Respect is often thought to reflect:

- beliefs;
- evaluative judgements;
- commitments;
- dispositions of attitude and behaviour towards the person who is being respected.

Reflection

1. Think of a situation where you feel that another person has been treated with disrespect. Identify what form/s of respect were disregarded. Was it someone's authority or position that was ignored or undermined? Was it the attitude of a person towards another that seemed disrespectful? Were any rules or boundaries broken? Was it a combination of some or all of these factors?

2. Think again. Can you identify why the person was treated this way?

3. In your view, how should this situation have been handled? What should have happened?

The principle of respect for persons

As children we are generally taught to respect significant others such as parents, elders, teachers, people 'in authority' but, as we get older, we may come to develop a deeper understanding of the value of respect for other people, connected with their feelings, rights and differing opinions. We may have great respect for some people based purely on a positive assessment of their merits or social standing and consider them exemplary, or lose respect for others, dependent on judgements of whether they are truly worthy of our respect. Alternatively, we may come to believe that all people are worthy of respect, irrespective of whether they display any merits, because of their humanity, as unique individuals and simply because they are persons.

Respect for persons as persons should also be distinguished from respect for persons in particular roles or based only on the positive assessment of the merits of an individual. Respect for persons is not simply about 'liking' or even 'agreeing with' someone or something and, although it involves an emotional response, it is not merely about sentiment but requires a corresponding disposition to respond and act respectfully towards the object of respect, i.e. the person. Equally, respect is more than just respectful behaviour, as simply to behave in a way that appears respectful, without valuing that respect, is deceitful. Thus the motive behind your show of respect for another person is as morally important as knowing how to act respectfully. For example, being careful not to use any racially inappropriate language while caring for an Asian family because you do not want to be caught breaching race discrimination laws is not sufficient motive to be considered respectful. In this case, your fear of legal recrimination is more about self-interest than the value of respect for others, even though it is showing respect for the authority of the law. The motive for your action should come from the value you attributed to them as persons with equal rights to respect and because you believe all individuals are unique and valued members of society. Dillon (1992, cited by Dillon, 2007, Sect. 1.2) identifies what he calls 'care respect', which encompasses this belief that persons have a unique value deserving of special concern and care. Thus, respect for persons at the very least involves:

- a belief in the value of persons as individuals and as members of society;
- treating people in the manner in which you expect to be treated;
- showing consideration for another person's feelings and interests;
- an attitude demonstrating that you value another person.

Many of the ordinary rules and judgements of common social morality (our ordinary shared moral beliefs) presuppose respect for persons as a fundamental foundation of all other moral duties and obligations. In this way, the principle of respect for persons can be considered to be universal. In other words, it should not have any national, cultural, legal or economic boundaries. This is also evident in much of the discussion of values and ethics associated with health and care practice, where respect for persons is seen as an essential guiding principle that underpins all others (Banks, 2006; Beauchamp and Childress, 2001; Seedhouse, 1998). For example, if you act according to the principle that it is wrong to harm another then this will, in part, be based on the fact that you value their humanity and them as a unique individual, with feelings and interests that should not be violated.

RESPECT, DIGNITY AND PRIVACY IN PRACTICE

Dignity

Respect for persons is also one of the defining attributes of the concept of dignity (see Figure 2.3) and both give rise to other duties, including the duty of confidentiality and the respect you should have for other people's privacy. We will come back to look at confidentiality in more detail in Chapter 4 on 'Trust, confidentiality and truth-telling'.

> **Dignity**
>
> Dignity consists of many overlapping aspects including respect, privacy, auton-omy and self-worth. The definition of dignity used by the Social Care Institute for Excellence (SCIE)(2006, p.1) is:
>
> > a state, quality or manner worthy of esteem or respect; and (by extension) self-respect. Dignity in care, therefore, means the kind of care, in any setting, which supports and promotes, and does not undermine, a person's self-respect regardless of any difference.

Figure 2.3 Definition of dignity

The next activity requires you to think carefully about respect for persons, dignity and privacy in your practice.

Case study

Barbara

You are visiting your mother, Barbara, who is 82 years old. She is dependent on a wheelchair for mobility and has recently chosen to move into a residential home as she was finding it increasingly difficult to cope on her own (you are her only close relative and live some distance away). When you arrive she is sitting in the main living room. She is wearing clothes you do not recognise and her hair appears to have been 'blown dry' (for as long as you can remember she has always had a weekly 'shampoo and set'). She is normally chatty, cheer-ful and pleased to see you but today she is tearful and agitated.

You ask a member of staff if there is a room where you can take your mother to talk (she shares a room with two other women and one is already resting in the room). They say that all the other rooms are occupied and suggest you simply move to the other corner of the sitting room away from the television. They seem to stay nearby as if to hear what you are saying to each other.

Your mother reveals tearfully that when she was taking her daily bath that morning, one of the male care assistants had entered the bathroom to get a commode and trolley that were stored in the corner of the room. The female member of staff assisting your mother had made light of the incident, saying light-heartedly, 'Barbara, fancy your "boyfriend" coming to see you in the bath'. Your mother is obviously upset but says the young woman meant no malice and urges you not to make a fuss.

1. What issues are there to be considered here in relation to respect, dignity and privacy? As well as specific aspects of care practice, think also about other features, such as the care environment.

2. What would you do differently in this situation?

3. Having thought about the importance of maintaining respect and dignity in this case, make a list of ways in which you can practise to ensure that your care respects individuals and maintains their dignity. Discuss your list with a colleague and add any new ideas that emerge from your conversation.

4. Now find out whether there is a dignity policy in your work environment. If there is, read it and make notes of the key principles to be observed in your workplace.

Self-respect, self-worth and dignity can all too easily be undermined by the attitudes and approaches of others. Research with older people has highlighted the ways in which carers can reinforce the negative aspects of their situation, such as their dependency and fragility, which can make them feel insignificant and unrecognised as individuals, and which, in turn, compromises their self-respect and dignity (SCIE, 2006). Older people use strategies to maintain a sense of self-worth and meaning in their lives, such as focusing on simple pleasures and maintaining their sense of normality, feeling needed and having connections with their families and remembering their previous life and achievements. However, these can easily be either positively reinforced and supported or unfortunately undermined by the practice of health and social care workers in their everyday interactions with people in their care (SCIE, 2006).

Privacy

Respect for persons in the case study above is not only concerned with dignity and self-worth. It is also closely associated with respect for Barbara's privacy. Privacy is again a concept that can be looked at in a number of ways. You may think about it from a very practical viewpoint such as, for example, maintaining privacy by drawing curtains when meeting patients' hygiene needs or knocking on doors before entering cubicles. Alternatively, you could identify with the underlying moral principles or values related to maintaining privacy, such as establishing a relationship of trust, the importance of respecting the person, treating them as an individual and promoting and supporting their independence. All of these perspectives are important for, if you are to develop and enhance your practice, you need to be able to think not only about what you should do but also the value associated with practising in a certain way, i.e. why you should do this. Woogara (2004, p.34) identifies four interrelated characteristics essential to understanding privacy of the person, namely:

- respect for the person;
- privacy of the body;
- privacy of one's space and territory;
- having control and choice of one's surroundings.

You should have been able to recognise violation of all of these aspects of a person's privacy in the case study and identified different approaches that would demonstrate respect for Barbara as a person and to provide care in a way that maintains her individuality and protects and preserves her privacy as a person. It is often in the very fundamental aspects of care, such as meeting hygiene needs, that dignity, respect for the individual and their privacy can be most at risk, particularly if care becomes routinised and you underestimate the aspects of care that are taken for granted, which can pose real threats to an individual's self-esteem and well-being.

The reality for patients and service users requiring care in hospitals, care homes or in their own homes is that they will inevitably expose themselves to practitioners and carers in ways, both physically and personally, that would not occur in their normal everyday lives. Sleeping in rooms with other people, sharing communal bathing and toilet facilities, using commodes with only the 'protection' of a flimsy curtain, discussing personal thoughts, feelings and intimate information with relative strangers in the process of assessment and diagnosis are all examples that can compromise a person's privacy and challenge their ability to maintain their personal self-respect and dignity. I will always remember the humiliation I felt at 18 years' old when, on a busy orthopaedic ward following surgery, I was expected to use a bedpan without any curtains at the end of the bed because this was the norm and I was told that 'anyway the bed cradle would act as a screen' even though I could clearly see the patients opposite me. I would hope that such practice would now be seen as totally unacceptable. However, it is easy to imagine situations where practitioners become desensitised to some of the expectations placed on patients and service users in the delivery of their care. There will inevitably be times where total privacy cannot be maintained. However, you must be able to justify any compromise of privacy, both on practical grounds and in terms of the service user's moral right to privacy. It is essential that you take responsibility for safeguarding the privacy and dignity of patients and service users in your delivery of care.

How can privacy and dignity be protected and promoted?

Research evidence

In 2007 the Healthcare Commission published the results of a survey of over 80,000 adult inpatients, which highlighted continuing concerns related to respect and dignity (Healthcare Commission, 2007). These included:

Just under one third (30%) of patients who were admitted to hospital as an emergency said that they shared a sleeping area such as a room or bay with a member of the opposite sex when they were first admitted. For respondents who were moved to another ward, this proportion then falls to 16%. About one in 10 patients (11%) who had a planned admission to hospital said that they shared a sleeping area such as a room or bay with a member of the opposite sex when they were first admitted to hospital.

Seventy per cent of patients said that they 'always' had enough privacy when discussing their condition or treatment on the ward and a further 22% said that they 'sometimes' had enough privacy. Most patients (88%) had enough privacy when being treated or examined.

Just over half of respondents (52%) said they were 'definitely' involved as much as they wanted to be in decisions about their care and treatment, with 37% saying they were involved 'to some extent'...the percentage of patients saying they were not as involved as much as they wanted to be (was) 11%... (79%) said they were given the right amount of information about their treatment or condition but 21% of patients said that they were given too little information ... the percentage of patients who said they were 'always' treated with respect and dignity is 78%. (Healthcare Commission, 2007)

Ensuring that privacy and dignity are protected and promoted is about far more than simply separating men and women in care environments (as identified in the research evidence extract above). Your attitude and approach to the way you deliver care are as much or more important than the environment itself and are everyone's responsibility. It is therefore essential that you are aware of the various circumstances in which a service user's privacy and dignity may be infringed and that you practise the knowledge, skills and values that will enable you to practise with sensitivity. Also, if you are serious about the importance of respect for persons in your care and their dignity then it is essential that you do not get lulled into the false sense of security provided by simply claiming to follow routines, protocols and guidelines. Observing these is only the first step to being committed to seeing, understanding and knowing the value of respect for others and to prevent behaviour and attitudes that degrade, devalue and humiliate individuals in your care. From the findings of the research conducted in the 'Dignity and the older European adult project' (2004), Tadd (2007) has identified several aspects essential to 'Dignity-enhancing care' (see Figure 2.4).

Dignity-enhancing care

- Promotes autonomy and individuality
- Engenders respect
- Involves effective communication
- Encourages involvement and participation
- Ensures privacy
- Empowers rather than humiliates
- Maintains personal identity.

Accessed via the Older People National Service Framework website at **www. wales.nhs.uk/sites3/docmetadata.cfm?orgid=439&id=76216** (accessed 9 January 2008)

Figure 2.4 Dignity-enhancing care (taken from Dr Win Tadd's conference presentation 'Dignity matters: A focus on the treatment of older people' for the National Service Framework for Older People Conference held on 22 January 2007)

One example of government policy and guidance that has a commitment to changing practice and attitudes and to promoting new ways of working is the *Essence of care* (DoH, 2003a) which aimed to embed good person-centred practice into the care of NHS patients (although its principles are also relevant to other care sectors). The benchmarking process outlined in the *Essence of care* claims:

> to help practitioners to take a structured approach to sharing and comparing practice, enabling them to identify the best and to develop action plans to remedy poor practice.
>
> (DoH, 2003a, p.1)

It is organised around ten key themes or 'benchmarks'. Figure 2.5 shows the factors that were identified, in consultation with patients, carers and professionals, as important to privacy and dignity. Although the benchmarks give broad areas of best practice related to each of the key factors, you need to think one stage further to identify specific practice examples that will meet each benchmark. For example, how might you practise to ensure that 'patients feel they matter all the time'? Or, what sort of manner should be used to ensure that 'communication between staff and patients respects their individuality'?

Patient-focused Outcome 1 'Patients benefit from care that is focused upon respect for the individual'. Taken from *Essence of care* (DoH, 2003a)	
Factor	Benchmark of best practice
Attitudes and behaviour	Patients feel that they matter all the time
Personal world and personal identity	Patients experience care in an environment that actively encompasses individual values, beliefs and personal relationships
Personal boundaries and space	Patients' personal space is actively promoted by all staff
Communicating with staff and patients	Communication between staff and patients takes place in a manner which respects their individuality
Privacy of patients – confidentiality of patient information	Patient information is shared to enable care, with their consent
Privacy, dignity and modesty	Patients' care actively promotes their privacy and dignity, and protects their modesty
Availability of an area for complete privacy	Patients and carers can access an area that safely provides privacy
Privacy = freedom from intrusion **Dignity = being worthy of respect**	

Figure 2.5 Benchmarks for privacy and dignity

Discussion activity

1. Using the Benchmark Statement in Figure 5.2, create a simple audit tool that could be used in your workplace to assess and evaluate practice in relation to one of the factors identified as important to respecting individuals, their privacy and maintaining their dignity. One way of doing this would be to write down your chosen key factor and benchmark, e.g. 'Privacy, dignity and modesty', and then create a list of related practices that would demonstrate achievement of the corresponding benchmark. You should have some ideas that you can take from your list created in response to Barbara's case study.

2. It would help if you could discuss your list with a group of practitioners and refine your audit tool.

To check and supplement your tool, you can refer back to the *Essence of care. Patient-focused benchmarks for clinical governance* document (DoH, 2003a) and look at the section for Privacy and dignity and their indicators for best practice identified by patients, carers and professionals and their current practice examples.

Practice notes

Practice to promote respect for persons and dignity (*adapted from Essence of care* (DoH, 2003a) and *Dignity in care practice guidance for adult services* (SCIE, 2006))

- Be self-aware and develop good communication and interpersonal skills.
- Act fairly, compassionately and sensitively.
- Ask individuals how they would prefer to be addressed, i.e. first name, surname, family name, etc.
- Ask for consent to share information with other carers.
- Where possible, orientate individuals to their environment including information about quiet areas, privacy and confidentiality.
- Take account of personal preferences, lifestyle choices and cultural factors when assessing their needs and providing support for care.
- Ensure people receive care or treatment in a dignified way that does not embarrass, humiliate or expose them; this includes the way information is exchanged at the bedside or in other communal environments.
- Don't make assumptions about appropriate standards of hygiene or appearance for individuals and provide support to maintain appearance to their level of expectation, e.g. hair, standards of

dress, etc. (for example, just because you shower every morning does not mean they should).

- Maintain confidentiality of personal and treatment information.
- Particular care is needed to maintain privacy when using interpreters; individuals may prefer to use a family member or the same interpreter on each occasion.
- Demonstrate respect for personal belongings such as, for example, access to individuals' own clothing, and privacy of personal space such, as for example, knocking on doors before entering rooms, using ways to prevent being disturbed when providing care at the bedside such as signs for curtains.
- Provide areas for private conversations, needs assessment, phone calls, etc.
- Enable individuals to personalise and make choices about their living environment, particularly in care homes.
- Be confident to challenge the negative attitudes of others.

THE MORAL DUTY OF RESPECT FOR PERSONS

Much of the contemporary discussion of respect for persons is most often accredited to the work of an eighteenth-century German philosopher, Immanuel Kant, who put respect for persons at the very centre of his moral theory. His original writings are complex and open to misinterpretation but it is worth highlighting some of the key points from his work that are relevant to the value of respect for persons in care practice.

Kant argued that all people are bearers of fundamental rights and that persons have an absolute dignity that is independent of rank or merit and must always be respected. Thus, persons have absolute value, unconditional and incomparable worth and exist as 'ends in themselves', in contrast to things that are valuable merely as a means to an end or as objects of affection. This value is common to all people and is concerned, not with being human beings *per se* (i.e. in a genetic sense), but with our humanity and the associated possession of the special features that make us distinctively human, including the capacities of 'reason and freedom of will', i.e. the ability for self-directed rational behaviour and to choose and follow our own moral goals. We will come back to some of these ideas in the discussion of respect for autonomy in Chapter 3. Thus, Kant believed that we should always act in ways that treat humanity as an end in itself, never merely or exclusively as a means to another person's ends.

If you think about this statement, you should be able to recognise that there is something intuitively wrong in treating human beings as merely instruments to achieve our own goals. An extreme example of this would be slavery. However, this does not totally rule out using people for our own purposes and we do this on a regular basis. Remember that we often treat people as a means to an end; for example, when I employ a plumber to fix my central heating, I am using him as a means to my own ends or purpose. What is important, however, is that I am not treating him merely as a means to my own ends because, in employing him, we both enter freely into a 'contract' (in this instance, involving payment). It is as much in the plumber's interests as mine that I employ him to do the job. He is able to make choices as to whether or not he wants to do this work or something else, he can influence when he is available to do the work, how much it will cost, etc. The same could be said of any person employed to provide a service, paid or voluntary, including care workers, as they have all chosen to enter into their role and with some purpose of their own. On the other hand, a slave is treated as a mere means to someone else's ends, they are generally not free to make choices about how they live their life and their main sole purpose is to fulfil another person's wishes and commands.

One example of the notion of 'using people as a means to an end' can be seen in health care when human research subjects are recruited to participate in trials for the testing of, for example, a new drug or treatment, as they are obviously being used for the potential benefit of others. However, this may be morally permissible if they have chosen and consented to participation. Some may get involved in research trials for altruistic reasons, i.e. their contribution to improving treatments for others and society; others will do it for their own benefits, including financial reward; or they may have both motives. In either case, they have not been used merely as a means to another's ends, they also had a purpose to their involvement and a choice as to whether or not they participated. The difficulties come in deciding whether or not they made their decision freely, whether the necessary conditions for informed choice and consent have been met, such as the provision of sound information and how voluntary their 'volunteering' may be. For example, offering money to participants is inevitably going to be more attractive to the less well-off members of society and this could be seen as manipulating their decision-making in such a way that they could not refuse. All of these aspects of achieving informed choice and consent relate closely to the principle of respect for autonomy, as you will see in Chapter 3. There are obviously rigorous guidelines for the ethical approval and conduct of medical research, for example, the Research Governance Framework for Health and Social Care (DoH, 2005c). However, the application of these rules and guidelines still depends on the moral integrity and values of the people conducting and participating in research.

Due respect for humanity

What Kant also required was not just a mere sense of respect for others but that, morally speaking, you should act with due respect for humanity. On this basis, you should develop and foster an attitude of due respect rather than simply a 'feeling' of respect. This is particularly pertinent to a value-based approach to caring for others. We owe persons respect simply because they are persons, regardless of whether we like them, they are useful to us or even if they have wronged us. Think about the value of respect for persons as you consider the following case study, 'Alfred in Accident and Emergency'.

Case study

Alfred in Accident and Emergency

Gemma is a health care assistant. She usually works in a medical ward but she has been sent to cover the evening shift in Accident and Emergency. Alfred, an elderly man, is brought in by ambulance; he is unkempt and dishevelled and smells strongly of alcohol. His clothes are stained with urine. He is well known to the locals; he is homeless and has been living on the streets for several years. Some passers-by called the ambulance when they saw him fall down a small flight of steps. Following initial assessment, it is established that he has no serious injuries but he has grazes on his hands and a small cut on his forehead. He is to be kept in overnight for observation. Staff usually take this opportunity to provide basic hygiene and clean clothes. Gemma is asked to wash Alfred's hands and face and to stay with him until a registered nurse is available to suture the cut. However, he has become extremely vocal, is swearing and cursing at any member of staff that goes near him and he is disturbing other patients and relatives. As she enters the cubicle, Alfred hurls verbal abuse at her and, when she offers to wash the blood from his hands and face and to get him some clean clothes, Alfred pushes her away forcefully.

Gemma starts to think that she's drawn the short straw. She doesn't see why she should subject herself to Alfred's vile language and abuse and if that's the way he feels and he doesn't want to be helped, then why should she bother? It is Alfred's choice after all.

1. What are your initial feelings about this case? Should Alfred's desire to be left alone be respected? Provide a justification for your answer.

2. Can a person forfeit their right to be respected? If so, give some examples of your reasoning.

This is an example where the desire to provide care and act in what you believe to be a person's best interests can come into conflict with duties arising from respect for them as persons, a conflict made more complex in this case by the individual's behaviour. Gemma appears to feel that Alfred's behaviour is unacceptable and it is true that there are limits to what you should have to endure in providing care, particularly as you too are deserving of respect as an individual. However, in these kinds of situations, it is not the case that the patient no longer deserves any respect for their humanity or as a person, even if they have quite different interpretations of what is in their best interests to yours. You may have identified that Gemma had obligations to ensure (as far as possible) Alfred's safety while in hospital, although this does not extend to insisting that he washes and changes his clothing. You may also have considered whether Alfred was capable of understanding what was in his best interests at this time and whether he was in full control of his decision-making and behaviour, particularly if he was under the influence of alcohol. This links to the discussion of competence and capacity in personal or individual autonomy in Chapter 3, but may also raise questions of how we define 'persons' when we talk about the value of respect for persons and those deserving of respect.

Defining the 'person'

One distinction that is important to the debate surrounding respect for persons and humanity is whether the terms 'human being' and 'person' are synonymous. There are two common interpretations of the term 'human life' or 'human being'. Firstly, it cannot be denied that a human being is a member of the species *Homo sapiens*; this has genetic, biological and scientific relevance. However, when we refer to the value of human life we are meaning much more than a preference for our own species. What is often intended when we talk about the value of the 'human being' is consideration of what makes them a 'person'. Recognition as a 'person' is significant in society because it lies at the centre of many debates about the status, respect, rights and treatments that are obligatory to different types of living beings. Thus, the notion of respect for persons inevitably requires some definition of what is meant by 'persons' although this in itself can be contentious. For example, in philosophy and applied ethics, the definition of 'person' generally excludes human beings who are incapable of certain kinds of thought like, for example, embryos, fetuses, newborn infants or adult humans that lack the capacity to reason. There are many definitions of 'person' put forward in the literature that incorporate a wide and varied range of defining characteristics and the recognition of status as a person is known as 'personhood'.

Definitions

One significant definition of persons comes again from the philosopher Kant, who makes some assumptions about 'persons' being rational beings, capable of rational thought and self-determination, where rationality relates to being able to give reasons for your actions and self-determination means being able to make decisions and act according to your own choices and desires (Banks, 2006, p.29). Kant also saw persons as having the ability to determine their own moral law, i.e. the moral rules and obligations that guide their actions, and that it is this that makes them intrinsically valuable. Other common characteristics that feature in definitions of the 'person' include:

- possessing human genetic material;
- having potential for human development;
- the necessity of birth;
- personal identity;
- individuality;
- presence of self-concept and self-awareness;
- a sense of self that persists through time;
- someone capable of valuing their own existence;
- development of communication and language;
- the ability to reason;
- reflective capacity.

Further definitions of persons and personhood can be seen in Figure 2.6.

Discussion activity

1. Can you identify any potential problems in your practice if the definitions of persons identified in Figure 2.6 were to be used in judgements of who (or what kinds of people) should be worthy of respect?

2. Make a list of examples where there may be conflict with the above definitions of persons.

3. Talk to friends or colleagues about what features in your list. Do they agree? If not, what are the reasons for their differences of opinion?

For example, these definitions are commonly used as just one of the arguments to justify the act of abortion, i.e. if the fetus is not capable of reasoning and self-awareness then it is not a person. It then follows, n this argument, that if the fetus is not a person, it is not deserving of the same level of respect as the 'fully fledged' human being. Therefore, on this account, termination of pregnancy is morally permissible.

Singer (1993, p.86) refers to Fletcher's (1972) 'indicators of humanhood', seeing these to be synonymous with personhood, i.e:

- self-awareness;
- self-control;
- a sense of the future;
- a sense of the past;
- the capacity to relate to others;
- concern for others;
- communication;
- curiosity.

Locke (1690, cited by Gillon, 1986, p.51) defined a 'person' as:

a thinking intelligent being that has reason and reflection and can consider itself as itself, the same thinking being in different times and place; which is inseparable from thinking and as it seems to me essential to it.

Warren (1973) includes in her definition of the 'person' possession of:

- consciousness ... (particularly) the capacity to feel pain;
- reasoning (the developed capacity to solve new and relatively complex problems);
- self-motivated activity;
- the capacity to communicate ... on indefinitely many possible topics;
- the presence of self-concepts, and self-awareness.

According to Lockwood (1985 p.10), a person:

must have the capacity for reflective consciousness and self-consciousness. It must have, or at any rate have the ability to acquire, a concept of itself, as a being with a past and a future.

Figure 2.6 Some definitions of persons and personhood

If you hold the view that persons are identified simply by 'being human', i.e. the possession of human genetic material, then this would suggest that some of the practices that society already endorses are immoral such as, for example, termination of pregnancy (which, of course, does concur with some people's views). However, you can see in the definitions in Figure 2.6 that persons can be defined as beings capable of having interests that other living things do not, or cannot, have, which suggests that it is these capacities that cause us to attribute value to persons. But, if you believed that the value of people is based purely in their capacity to be rational, self-determining, able to value themselves and to reason, then there could be a significant number of people to whom any duty of respect would not be owed, such as, for example, those with complex learning disabilities or severe mental health problems or the older person with some form of dementia. To simply judge who is owed respect on the basis of such capacities does not sit well with our intuitions about valuing and respecting humanity. Also, there may be many beings who are not rational and self-conscious (thus not fulfilling these criteria of personhood) and yet are capable of experiencing pleasure and suffering and to whom we would still attribute value and respect. Singer (1993, p.101) refers to these as 'conscious beings'. Many non-human animals may well fall into this category but it could also include, for example, newborn infants and those in persistent vegetative states. In recent years it has been argued that moral respect ought also to be extended to things other than persons, such as non-human living things and the natural environment. Thus, valuing conscious life and the very fact that someone is human is as important as valuing 'personhood' as defined above and emphasises that respect and dignity relate to every human regardless of their capacities, hence why we have talked here about respect for humanity as well as persons.

However, it is this notion of personhood, and the way it is defined and interpreted, which can cause dilemmas in practice. This arises from judgements about an individual's competence and capacity to be autonomous in their decisions about their own care, and your duties to act in a person's best interests and protect them from harm. Such dilemmas can give rise to allegations of paternalism. Paternalism occurs when you act in a way that overrides a person's own autonomous choices or preferences on the basis that you believe you are acting in their best interests, i.e. to benefit or avoid harm to the individual. Capacity and competence are particularly relevant to issues related to individual choice and consent, and in formal prescriptive definitions of legal capacity or personhood such as those defined in the Mental Capacity Act 2005. The notions of capacity and competence are explored further in Chapter 3 on autonomy and respect for autonomy.

Although defining persons is not straightforward, the value of 'respect for persons' is a starting point for good morality because it accepts the basic premise that other people matter and this is an important value in a society-based context. Humans do not and have never lived as isolated beings and, consequently, if people are destined to live together mutual respect should be a fundamental principle. Downie and Telfer (1967, cited in Hill, 1998) characterise respect as 'valuing and cherishing persons for what they are'. This encapsulates an important view in the care environment as it allows for difference, without a value judgement being placed upon that difference. From this, the fundamental duty to respect others should generally be independent of a person's personal characteristics and be afforded to all humans equally, regardless of their merit or ability.

The value of respect for persons is at the centre of the Department of Health White Paper *Valuing people: a new strategy for learning disability for the 21st century* (DoH, 2001b) and its subsequent reports. Although the focus of this paper is related to people with learning disabilities, the principles and good practice emerging as a result of this document (and a substantial amount of collaborative work between service users, their carers, families, statutory and non-statutory agencies and practitioners) are transferable to other client groups and care settings. Equally, regardless of your practice setting, you will inevitably meet people with learning disabilities, and their families and carers, as they may access the full range of health and social care services at some time.

Reading activity

Find and access the Valuing People website at: **http://valuingpeople. gov.uk/index.jsp**

This website provides the gateway to a wealth of important government documents, research, service user and carer resources and evidence of implementation of good practice.

1. Locate the document *Valuing people: a new strategy for learning disability for the 21st century* White Paper (DoH, 2001b) and its subsequent reports.

2. Make notes on the key principles identified in this White Paper which apply equally to all people with learning disabilities and their carers.

3. What are the implications of the key values in the *Valuing people* White Paper for your practice?

From the Resources area of the Valuing People website you can access a specific section related to 'Person-centred approaches'.

4. What are the five key features of person-centred planning?

5. Read at least one example where person-centred planning has been put into practice.

As with any aspect of health and social care, evaluation and research play an important part in establishing and maintaining good practice.

Locate the research report by Robertson, J., Emerson, E., Hatton, C. and Elliott, J., *et al.* (2005) *The impact of person centred planning.* April 2005, Institute for Health Research, Lancaster University (this is available on the Valuing People website).

6. Summarise the key findings of this report. What are the advantages and challenges of person-centred planning?

CONCLUSION

In this chapter you have explored the value of respect for persons as a core value and, if this is properly understood and integrated into care, many of the other values will flow from it. Having respect for persons and their humanity facilitates a philosophy of care that promotes dignity for service users even in situations of great dependence. The importance placed on privacy in maintaining an individual's dignity and the need to develop care strategies that protect and promote privacy have been emphasised.

We have identified that respect for persons is associated with a number of other values such as valuing humanity, dignity and privacy. However, we have consciously separated out respect for persons and autonomy, as it is important that you recognise and remember that although they are inter-related they are also distinct. Respect for persons is a value that implies a broader set of obligations than simply respecting an individual's auton-omy, which has self-determination as its main focus. However, the value associated with respect for autonomy is important in today's health and care practice and gives rise to a number of guiding principles and proce-dural aspects of care such as, for example, the importance of service user and carer involvement, the notions of empowerment and self-advocacy and the requirements for informed choice and consent.

SUMMARY OF KEY POINTS
- The values of respect and dignity are fundamental to care practice.
- If respect is properly understood and integrated into care, many of the other values will flow from it.
- Having respect for persons and their humanity promotes the dignity of service users even in situations of great dependence.
- Dignity and privacy can easily be compromised if care becomes routinised, therefore you must be conscious in your practice of working in ways that protect and promote the privacy of the service user.

FURTHER READING

Department of Health (2001b) *Valuing people: a new strategy for learning disability for the 21st century*. London: The Stationery Office

Social Care Institute for Excellence (SCIE) (2006) *Practice guide for adult services 09: 'Dignity in care'*, November 2006. London: SCIE

Chapter 3

Autonomy and the Principle of Respect for Autonomy

Key themes

In this chapter you will:

- identify the distinction between being autonomous and the principle of respect for autonomy;

- define personal autonomy and identify and discuss the necessary conditions to be autonomous, including the notions of capacity and competence;

- examine duties and rules arising from respect for autonomy and their implications for practice;

- explore the notion of paternalism and reflect on care strategies that promote autonomy.

INTRODUCTION

Autonomy and the principle of respect for autonomy are, arguably, fundamental values both in daily life and in health and care practice. However, before we go any further, there is an important distinction to be made here. 'Being autonomous' is a condition or state of being usually associated with individuals (that we may attribute value to), whereas respect for autonomy is a guiding principle, i.e. a rule or obligation to act or practise with due respect for another person's autonomy. Obviously, to understand this principle you need first to explore what it means to be autonomous.

DEFINING AUTONOMY

Writing activity

1. Think about and write down all the words, phrases and ideas that come to mind when you think about autonomy. What does being autonomous mean to you? If it helps, do a spider diagram:

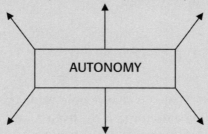

2. Look up 'autonomy' in a dictionary and add the definition to your 'mind map'.

3. Now talk to some relatives, friends and/or colleagues about what autonomy means to them.

4. Try writing your own definition of autonomy.

You may find that your list and definition have words and phrases that are similar to some of the things, such as the capacity to make choices and decisions, already discussed in Chapter 2 on respect for persons and defining persons. This is not surprising as autonomy and the principle of respect for autonomy are closely associated with respect for persons and the idea that if we value and respect people as individuals, then we should also respect their ability to make choices, determine their own life course and to be in control of their own lives without undue interference from others. Autonomy is inevitably important in cultures where all individuals are considered to be unique and valued members of society.

The word 'autonomy' is derived from the Greek word *autos* meaning 'self' and *nomos* meaning 'rule, governance or law'. Different writers give different accounts of autonomy, although most acknowledge that autonomy incorporates the capacity for self-determination or self-rule. Definitions of autonomy often include reference to terms such as:

- self-governance;
- independence;
- individuality;
- self-choice/individual choice;
- freedom/freedom of will;
- being one's own person.

Gerald Dworkin (1988, p.5), in his classic text *The theory and practice of autonomy*, reminds us that there are many different interpretations of the term 'autonomy'. It may be used to mean self-rule or liberty. It is often equated with dignity, integrity, individuality, responsibility, independence and is associated with the personal qualities of self-assertion, critical reflection and with having knowledge of one's own interests. However, he goes on to state that:

> the only features held constant ... are that autonomy is a feature of persons and that it is a desirable quality to have.
> (Dworkin, 1988, p.6)

What Dworkin alludes to here is that people value their autonomy; most people would see 'being autonomous' or having 'respect for individual's autonomy' as being desirable qualities or aims. Some reasons why we value autonomy are that:

- people are usually the best judge of what is good for them, so respecting their autonomous decisions will, on the whole, contribute to their happiness and well-being;
- being autonomous is part of human flourishing; people have a deep need to discover, create and express their own individual characters;
- value is attributed to persons and their unconditional worth.

Christman (2003, p.3) uses the term 'basic autonomy' to mean 'the minimal status of being responsible, independent and able to speak for oneself ... and free of manipulative, self-distorting influences'. This definition reflects the fact that most adults will be autonomous, except perhaps those who are suffering extremes of debilitating illness or from oppressive and constricting social constructs, contexts, practices or institutions. This is important to remember in the health and care context as you should always start from the assumption that a person has, at the very least, this basic autonomy, or is capable of being autonomous, unless there are strong justifiable reasons to think otherwise. Autonomy is not an all-or-nothing concept; it is a matter of degree and it is possible to be autonomous in some regards or at some times and not others. We assume that you would generally consider yourself to be autonomous yet you may well have experienced times when you felt your usual level of autonomy was compromised, as, for example, during illness.

In addition, being autonomous is usually associated with being an adult. However, there is a significant amount of research that considers children's developing ability to be autonomous and their rights to be involved in decisions that impact on them as individuals and their present and future lives. If you want to read more about this, a good place to start is with work by Priscilla Alderson, who writes passionately about making care decisions with children and their families (see Alderson and Montgomery, 1996; Alderson, 2000, 2002).

Formal definitions and key components of autonomy

> Individual autonomy is an idea that is generally understood to refer to the capacity to be one's own person, to live one's life according to reasons and motives that are taken as one's own and not the product of manipulative or distorting external forces.
>
> (Christman, 2003, p.1)
>
> Autonomy when applied to individuals refers to the ability of a person to decide their own fate; the autonomous individual has the freedom and the ability to make decisions independently or to exercise choices for themselves.
>
> (Blakemore, 2003, p.257)
>
> Beauchamp and Childress (2001, p.58) define personal autonomy as:
>
> > self-rule that is free from both controlling interferences by others and from personal limitations that prevent meaningful choice, such as inadequate understanding.
>
> Gillon's (1986, p.60) definition has similar requirements, in that he states that autonomy is:
>
> > the capacity to think, decide and act on the basis of such thought and decision freely and independently and without let or hindrance.

Figure 3.1 Some formal definitions of autonomy

There are at least four elements relevant to autonomy that are implied by the definitions in Figure 3.1. These are:

- the value of respect for persons;
- the ability to be self-governing and being able to determine one's personal goals, preferences and desires;
- the capacity or competence to make choices or decisions based on our deliberation and reason;
- the freedom to make choices for oneself and then to act on these.

Imaginative exercise

Imagine you are on a weight-reducing diet and you have been really pleased with your weight loss so far. However, today is turning out to be a particularly stressful day at work, so when you go for coffee you cannot resist buying a Danish pastry and a chocolate bar. You feel you deserve them given the morning you have had but, once you have eaten them, you feel guilty and angry with yourself and wish you hadn't let yourself down in this way.

1. Was choosing to eat the Danish pastry and chocolate an autonomous decision?

2. How might you explain your decision and actions to another person?

Many of us may have been in situations like this and, perhaps, deciding to eat one cake or bar of chocolate will not be a tragedy as far as the diet is concerned. However, whether or not you said you were autonomous in this decision-making helps to illustrate some of the complexities in understanding autonomy. We would expect that you consider yourself to be an autonomous adult and that, in making a choice here, even if it was for cake and chocolate, you might have felt that you were still acting autonomously as this was your own individual decision. Some concept of basic or minimal autonomy might well concur with this view. However, in the scenario above, it appears that this might not, on reflection, have been your truly autonomous decision given that you feel guilty and angry and have regrets for your actions. It is as if you are reasoning that your initial actions succumbed to some compulsions or influences, such as the satisfaction of basic desires for pleasure and comfort, which do not agree with your ultimate, higher-order aims to lose weight or eat a healthy diet.

Gillon (1986, p.61) helps us to understand a number of components of autonomy that are relevant here when he describes three types of autonomy:

- autonomy of thought;
- autonomy of will;
- autonomy of action.

Thinking about each of these should help you to recognise that a person's autonomy may be compromised in one or all of these areas.

Autonomy of thought

Autonomy of thought includes the wide range of intellectual skills that encompass the ability to think for oneself when deliberating about choices, desires, preferences and wants, believing things and making decisions like, for example, your conscious and reasoned decision to lose weight.

Autonomy of will

Autonomy of will (autonomy of intention) is the freedom to decide to do things based on your deliberations and intentions, i.e. your 'will-power'. For example, you can decide not to eat a chocolate bar despite the powerful desire to do so. However, autonomy of will may be diminished by a number of influences, either internal such as hunger or in other cases disease or addiction to drugs, or external, such as threats or manipulation.

Autonomy of action

Autonomy of action is acting for oneself; being able to act on the basis of one's autonomous thought and will. For example, a person with paralysis may have autonomy of thought but will be restricted in their autonomy of action because they are unable to act without the assistance of others.

Each of these forms of autonomy, i.e. of thought, will and action, requires some basis in reasoning – the ability to deliberate and think about options and choices and to establish a reason for the decision or action (although the quality of, or types of, reasons may differ between individuals, which is important to remember when considering the choices made by service users and in cases of determining competence).

Dworkin's (1988) account of autonomy highlights the need for individuals to have the capacity to reflect upon their preferences, desires and wishes and to change these in the light of higher-order desires. A person is said to act autonomously when they act on the desires they have decided to endorse (based in reflection), and when their decision is not the result of manipulation, coercion or other controlling influences. So, to go back to the imaginary cake and chocolate example, it appears that you had made a conscious and deliberate choice to lose weight and that this was your principal aim. It is not that this desire is better in itself (i.e. wanting to lose weight or eat healthier food is obviously or always better than eating cake and chocolate), it is the fact that you have reasoned and chosen this as your primary desire or preference. However, on this occasion you may have given way to some compulsions or 'controlling' influences, such as tiredness, stress, hunger and a basic desire for comfort. It is unlikely in this case that you were coerced, i.e. threatened or forced. However, you may have been subject to some external manipulating influences such as, for example, the positioning of chocolate and cakes (rather than fruit) close to the till point where you have to wait for your coffee or seeing 'special offers' if you buy the two items together, etc. You should also note that this does not mean that you lack autonomy altogether, just that your autonomy has been compromised temporarily in this particular aspect or decision.

These accounts of autonomy, which include reference to making choices on the basis of reflection on, and ordering of, our desires and preferences and being free from (or having the ability to resist) distorting or controlling influences, are particularly relevant in the context of health promotion and practice aimed at helping individuals to review and change their health behaviours.

Reflection

Think of one aspect of your practice where you may be expected to support an individual to change their health behaviour. This could include supporting someone with smoking cessation, advising a parent in the provision of a healthier diet for their child, working with someone who drinks excessive amounts of alcohol, encouraging safer sex practices, introducing exercise regimes following a myocardial infarction (heart attack). If you cannot think of an example from practice, you could reflect on a change you may have tried to make at home like, for example, encouraging everyone to eat five pieces of fruit and vegetables a day.

1. Would you consider the person/people you were working with to be fully autonomous? Explain your answer. Think about the accounts of autonomy presented by Gillon (1986) and Dworkin (1988).

2. What challenges have you faced in advising or supporting the individual?

3. Was their autonomy compromised in any way? What kinds of influences could interfere with their autonomy?

In completing this exercise you should have started to identify that there are number of factors or conditions that affect whether or not an individual can be autonomous in their choices, decision-making and actions.

NECESSARY CONDITIONS TO BE AUTONOMOUS

For an individual to be autonomous, i.e. to choose and act for themselves, at least two key components are required.

1. Competence to make choices, i.e. the individual is able to understand and think about their situation.
2. Freedom from overwhelming influences or interferences that would prevent an individual making choices for themselves.

Some of the influences on the person making a choice will be internal to the individual, for example, having the ability to reason; others will be external, for example, the environment and the effect of others, including family, friends and carers, that can impact on an individual's decision-making.

Reflection

Think about an important decision that you have had to make in your personal life. It could be buying or renting a new property, buying a new car or an expensive piece of electrical equipment for your house, or something else that is of significant value to you.

1. What decision did you have to make? What options did you have?

2. What did you do to help you make a choice?

3. How long did it take from first identifying the need to reach a decision, for example, to complete the purchase?

4. Who else was involved in the decision-making? This may have included friends, relatives and strangers. In what ways did they influence your decision?

5. Did anything hinder your final decision-making?

6. Were you confident in the decision that you made? If not, explain why not.

Hopefully you will see from your reflections that being autonomous can be a complex activity, particularly where we are called upon to make important, unfamiliar or demanding choices outside of our normal day-to-day decision-making. Similar challenges confront patients and service users when they are faced with choices outside of their normal realm of decision-making or where the consequences of their decisions are potentially life-changing or life-threatening. Through completing this reflective exercise, you will have identified a number of factors or conditions that are necessary in order for an individual to be autonomous. These should include the following points:

Understanding
- Being able to understand the issues involved and being able to reflect and weigh them up – what may be referred to as having the competence or capacity to make choices and decisions, although this is difficult to determine and different standards of competence are often applied and required.

Information
- Having adequate information on which to base the decision (this need not be all available information but it should be sufficient to weigh up the pros and cons or the harms and benefits of a particular choice or action and its potential consequences).

Having choices
- – i.e. if individuals are being asked to choose then there must be real and meaningful options to choose from.

Deliberation
- Having the opportunity to deliberate – having time to reflect on choices and options and to check out understanding is important, particularly in new contexts or with unfamiliar decisions. A knee-jerk reaction is rarely an autonomous choice.

Voluntariness
- Being able to act voluntarily and to be free from untoward manipulation or coercion (threat) when making choices and decisions.

Environment
- Being in an environment that supports and fosters autonomy; the individual must believe that their autonomous choice will be facilitated, fostered and supported.

The opportunity to exercise choice.
- Having made a choice, the individual must be able to put that choice into action without fear of punishment or recrimination.

Influencing decisions

The role you play in the relationship with a service user is obviously an important external influence on their ability to be autonomous. You may feel that the likelihood of coercion or threat is minimal. Obviously, any form of threat will erode an individual's autonomy and it is possible that quite subtle forms of influence may be perceived as threatening by some service users and patients. For instance, if you give a service user a range of options but imply in some way that, if they do not choose a particular one, they may lose your support, care or concern, this may easily be perceived as a threat. The environment may also be threatening and not conducive to making decisions such as, for example, a clinical environment. It is also far too easy to manipulate a person's choice without using threat but still in ways that undermine their autonomy – a disapproving look, telling lies, withholding information about, for example, unpleasant side-effects. We will look at the value of truth-telling in Chapter 4.

However, not all influences distort autonomy. Influencing a person's choices through rational persuasion, with the intention of informing their decisions such as, for example, giving the evidence about the efficacy of a particular intervention or explaining the potential consequences of their actions (even when these may be unpleasant), appeals to reason rather than emotion. The requirements of informed choice and informed consent in health and care, where sufficient appropriate information must be given to make a reasoned decision, are based in the value placed on being autonomous and having control in your choices and decisions. But remember; too much information or confusing and conflicting information given without opportunity for discussion can also hinder a person's autonomy.

Having the freedom to make decisions

Being autonomous is therefore associated with an individual's ability to make their own self-determined choices, involves a degree of independence and the capacity to reason and to reflect on their desires and preferences in their decision-making. It also requires, to some extent, that each person has the freedom to make decisions about, express and act on their personal preferences, desires and goals. For example, if we said to you that you must spend all weekend reading and doing the exercises in this book as it would be in your best interests, you might well reply that you have other things planned and, anyway, how do we know what is right for you when in fact you learn best by doing small chunks of study over a period of time? You will inevitably base your decisions about our suggestion on a range of factors, including your past learning experiences, information guiding your learning (for example, advice from tutors and the learning outcomes in a course or module), the immediate relevance of the book to you at this time (for example, having an assignment that is due in on Monday that requires you to say something about your values in practice), other demands on your time such as family commitments that impact on your priorities for your weekend, etc. However, as an autonomous person, you are free to choose whether or not you heed our advice but, equally, in exercising that right to choose you also have to accept responsibility for your decision. The same applies in health and care. For example, the White Paper *Choosing health: making healthy choices easier* (DoH, 2004a) sets out the key principles for supporting the public to make healthier and more informed choices but also aims to encourage individuals to take responsibility for their health.

Being autonomous is also not about being self-centred and excessively individualistic or asocial, and consideration must be given to how your freedom to exercise your own autonomy impacts on that of others. Therefore, you may be justified in not respecting a person's autonomy if their action would result in significant harm to others. For example, as an adult, you are free to choose to drink any amount of alcohol you wish. However, if you then choose to drive while over the legal limit of alcohol we would be justified in trying to stop you because of the risk you would cause to other road users and pedestrians (and there would be legal penalties and possible restrictions of your future freedoms such as, for example, the removal of your driving licence or imprisonment if our warnings went unheeded). The legislation resulting in the ban on smoking in public places (perhaps more controversial than drink-driving because of those who see this as an infringement of liberties) was passed in order to restrict freedom of choice on the basis that individuals who smoke are 'free' to choose to take risks with their own health (all things considered) but should not be able to impose the potential harmful consequences of their choices on others. However, if we made moves to stop you driving or smoking, not on the basis of the risks to others, but because we felt it was in your best interests, we could be deemed to be acting paternalistically.

Paternalism

Paternalism only exists in actions that fail to respect a person's autonomy but are done with the intent of benefiting that person (or to prevent them being harmed). Thus, you would be acting paternalistically if the person is at least minimally autonomous and you either:

- prevent a person from acting or force them to act in a particular way, or do something to them without their consent, because it is in their best interests; or
- interfere with their autonomous decision-making by, for example, withholding information but, again, because it is for their own good.

Whether or not paternalism can ever be justified will depend upon the value placed on acting in someone's best interest versus the value placed on autonomy. Paternalism is more likely to be justified where an individual's autonomy is compromised, although decisions of this kind are highly contentious. For example, should doctors transfuse blood as a life-saving intervention in an emergency situation to an unconscious patient who is a Jehovah's Witness, in spite of their express advance directive that they do not consent to receiving blood? In the past, paternalism was common, with practitioners frequently providing care and interventions without adequate service user involvement in the decision-making process. However, it is now recognised to be a more controversial approach to practice and respect for service user preferences and choices has to be balanced with the degree of risk and harm that may result. We will explore this further in Chapter 5, 'Protection from harm and promoting independence'.

Generally the rule that follows from respect for persons is that you should accept and respect an individual's autonomous preferences and choices unless their actions will cause harm to others or if their autonomy is significantly compromised in some regard such that they are unable to make autonomous choices. This raises the issue of capacity or competence in individual autonomy and decision-making.

CAPACITY AND COMPETENCE

Anything that limits an individual's personal capacities to weigh up information and make choices will compromise their autonomy. Deliberation of whether or not a person has the capacity to be autonomous in decision-making raises discussion regarding their competence.

Reflection

1. What do you understand by the term 'competence'?

2. What factors may impact on a service user's or patient's competence?

3. Is competence an absolute, all-or-nothing phenomenon, i.e. is an individual either competent or not competent? Explain your answer.

Competence is not easy to define and yet it plays a major role in decisions about whether or not individuals are autonomous and should therefore have their own choices about their care respected. Part of the confusion is in the terminology used. Beauchamp and Childress (2001, p.70) define competence as 'the ability to perform a task'. Think about any task that you have competence to perform. You will recognise that it requires a level of knowledge or information, certain skills and personal and external resources. Remember the first time you rode a bike or drove a car. It would be very unlikely that you had competence from the outset but instead had to learn to complete the task. In this sense, competence should be viewed as being relative to the task to be performed or the decision to be made, so you may be competent to drive a car but not competent to ride a horse. Competence can also vary over time and be intermittent; you may no longer be able to speak French as fluently as you did in school because you have not used or practised that learning for some time. It may be refreshed to some degree when you visit France on holiday and then lost again as it is not a skill you need to use in your everyday life. In just the same ways, service users and patients may be competent in some regards but not others and their competence may change over time depending on a range of circumstances, including their mental or physical state, social determinants or context or the familiarity or unfamiliarity of a situation, task or decision.

Standards of competence in health and care often focus on an individual's capacities to make choices and are therefore closely associated with the qualities of being autonomous, including the ability to:

- understand and process information;
- reflect on preferences;
- make a judgement about the information in light of their personal values;
- communicate their intentions;
- be free from distorting influences, particularly those internal to the individual, such as impaired memory, addiction, some forms of mental illness.

The competence of individuals in health care is therefore often judged against their capacity or ability to understand an intervention (or task), to deliberate regarding its risks and benefits and to make a decision in light of these deliberations (Beauchamp and Childress, 2001, p.72). Beauchamp and Childress (2001, p.73) go on to present a range of inabilities that may be used to distinguish incompetence, which cluster according to three kinds of ability or skill (see Figure 3.2).

You will no doubt see a range of strategies used to judge competence of service users in your practice that will inevitably impact on the degree to which the service users are deemed to be autonomous and how far their wishes and preferences are acknowledged and respected. The law would generally assume adults to be competent unless proved otherwise, although an increasing gravity of the consequences of their decision may demand a higher level of competence. Inevitably, an individual's capacity in autonomous decision-making may be affected, for example, by mental illness, learning disability, dementia, brain injury or other

Type of ability or skill	Inabilities used to judge incompetence
Ability to state a preference (a weak standard)	1 Inability to express or communicate a preference or choice
Abilities to understand information and appreciate one's situation	2 Inability to understand one's situation and its consequences 3 Inability to understand relevant information
Abilities to reason about a consequential life decision (Standard 7 is the only one to restrict the acceptable outcomes of reasoning)	4 Inability to give a reason 5 Inability to give a rational reason 6 Inability to give risk/benefit-related reasons 7 Inability to reach a reasonable decision (as judged by a reasonable person's standard)

Figure 3.2 Inabilities used to judge incompetence (adapted from Beauchamp and Childress, 2001, p.73)

disease processes. Capacity may also be affected temporarily due, for example, to fear, pain or confusion. However, you should never assume that what affects one person will lead to the same level of incapacity in another. Care must also be taken when individuals appear to make what seems to you to be an irrational decision; this is where it is particularly important to see the situation through the service user's eyes and from their value position. What is right for you is not necessarily what is right for another and it may be a fine line between competence and incompetence when people appear to choose to make unreasonable, eccentric or unwise decisions.

Legislation relating to capacity in care practice

The values and duties surrounding capacity in care practice have been made clearer in the United Kingdom by the legal standards of capacity expressed in the Mental Capacity Act 2005, which came into force in April 2007. The Act is intended:

> to be enabling and supportive of people who lack capacity, not restricting or controlling of their lives. It aims to protect people who lack capacity to make particular decisions, but also to maximise their ability to make decisions, or to participate in decision-making, as far as they are able to do so.
> (Department for Constitutional Affairs, 2007, p.19)

The associated *Mental Capacity Act 2005 – Code of Practice* published in 2007 (Department for Constitutional Affairs, 2007) outlines in detail those people who have a formal duty to observe the Code, such as professionals and paid carers, people acting as attorneys or as deputies appointed by the Court of Protection, and how the statutory principles should be applied in practice. However, it also provides guidance for less formal carers, family and friends. You should find time to read the *Mental Capacity Act 2005 – Code of Practice*, if you have not already done so, as it is an excellent resource with a wealth of practice examples that will challenge and consolidate your understanding of the issues associated with the competence of service users and their participation in care decisions (see Figure 3.3).

Section 1 of the Mental Capacity Act sets out the five 'statutory principles' – the values that underpin the legal requirements in the Act:

The five statutory principles are:

1. A person must be assumed to have capacity unless it is established that they lack capacity.

2. A person is not to be treated as unable to make a decision unless all practicable steps to help him to do so have been taken without success.

3. A person is not to be treated as unable to make a decision merely because he makes an unwise decision.

4. An act done, or decision made, under this Act for or on behalf of a person who lacks capacity must be done, or made, in his best interests.

5. Before the act is done, or the decision is made, regard must be had to whether the purpose for which it is needed can be as effectively achieved in a way that is less restrictive of the person's rights and freedom of action.

Following the principles and applying them to the Act's framework for decision-making will help to ensure not only that appropriate action is taken in individual cases, but also to point the way to solutions in difficult or uncertain situations.

A person's capacity (or lack of capacity) refers specifically to their capacity to make a particular decision at the time it needs to be made.

Figure 3.3 Section 1 of the Mental Capacity Act (taken from the *Mental Capacity Act 2005 – Code of Practice* (DCA, 2007, p.19)

A DUTY OF RESPECT FOR AUTONOMY

It follows from our discussion of respect for persons and the value placed on being autonomous that respect for autonomy is one of the fundamental principles that should guide your interactions with service users and the care that you provide. Respecting autonomy in practice means, at the very least, that you acknowledge:

> a person's rights to hold views, to make choices, and to take actions based on [their] personal values and beliefs. Such respect involves respectful *action*, not merely a respectful *attitude*. It also requires more than non-interference in others' personal affairs.
>
> (Beauchamp and Childress, 2001, p.63)

In order to respect the autonomy of patients and service users you will need to:

- communicate effectively;
- help to develop or maintain their capacities for autonomous choice;
- provide relevant information at an appropriate level of understanding and in a medium suitable for the service user;
- support the development of necessary skills;
- enable individuals to make decisions voluntarily and freely;
- help to dispel fears and other conditions that could impede autonomous decision-making and action;
- ensure the environment is conducive to their decision making;
- be prepared to accept their choices and respect their decisions, including those to refuse or withdraw from treatment or intervention, whatever the outcome.

However, respecting autonomy is not just about agreeing with the wishes of others. It may also involve the creation or increase of their autonomy and using strategies to enable individuals to make reasoned choices. It is not about simply saying 'over to you' when there are difficult decisions to be made. Autonomy should be thought of more broadly, and concern for service user and patient welfare is, in itself, a central part of autonomy creation. Without advice, support and education, an individual may have little or no autonomy to exercise (Seedhouse, 1998, pp.182–3). The notions of advocacy (ensuring the voice of the service user is heard) and empowerment (developing individuals' skills and self-confidence) are valuable enabling strategies that can enhance respect of the individual and their autonomy in their care decisions. The increasing emphasis on choice and the 'recovery approach' in mental health practice (which includes developing resilience and recovery of hope and ambition for living full and purposeful lives and achieving choice and control for individuals and their families) also reflects the values of respect and dignity and respect for autonomy. There is insufficient scope in this textbook to do justice to these concepts at the level they deserve and you are advised to follow up this chapter by reading some of the additional sources listed at the end that relate to these specific areas of work.

The principle of respect for autonomy also supports many more specific moral rules for practice, such as respecting the privacy of others (which we have already addressed) and truth-telling, protecting confidentiality and informed consent, which we turn to in Chapter 4 in relation to the value of trust and trustworthiness.

One of the dilemmas for practitioners caring for others will always be how to reconcile concern for welfare with respect for autonomy when the two come into conflict: for example, when an older person is prone to falling but refuses support or use of mobility aids. In Chapter 4, we talk more about the need for the careful balancing of values to respect an individual's right to independence with protecting an individual from harm. Independence and the ability to live life according to one's own preferences, beliefs and choices are important values for human flourishing and well-being and in maintaining a good quality of life. What is important is that you do not take for granted or make assumptions about people's ability (or inability) to be autonomous or deny them the respect that humanity deserves.

CONCLUSION

This chapter has focused on the value of autonomy and demonstrates that respect for autonomy is fundamental to care practice. Being respected, having our views taken seriously, being able to express our individuality and being able to make, and act on, our own choices and decisions are important features of our everyday lives. It is these things that give us a sense of worth and a sense of self. It is therefore essential that you develop your practice in ways that show proper respect for the autonomy of service users, patients and clients. The activities in this chapter have provided you with the opportunity to examine your own approach to care and to think about strategies that would enable you to provide opportunities to support those in your care to be autonomous.

SUMMARY OF KEY POINTS
- The values of autonomy and respect of autonomy are fundamental to care practice.
- Respect for our individuality and autonomy contributes to our well-being, a sense of worth and a sense of self.
- 'Being autonomous' requires a number of conditions, including the capacity to determine your own goals, make choices and being free to act on the basis of our decisions.

- Being autonomous also means taking responsibility for our own choices and actions.
- Respect for autonomy includes developing care strategies to support and enable others to be autonomous, including strategies to foster self-advocacy and empowerment.

FURTHER READING

Adams, R. (2003) *Social work and empowerment*. Basingstoke: Palgrave

Bateman, N. (2000) *Advocacy skills for health and social care professionals*. London: Jessica Kingsley

Department for Constitutional Affairs (2007) *Mental Capacity Act 2005. Code of Practice*. Crown Copyright. London: The Stationery Office

Care Services Improvement Partnership (CSIP), Royal College of Psychiatrists (RCPsych) and Social Care Institute for Excellence (SCIE) (2007) *A common purpose: recovery in future mental health services*. Position Paper 8. London: SCIE. (This report is available in print and online at **www.scie.org.uk**)

Chapter 4

Trust, Confidentiality and Truth-telling

Key themes

In this chapter you will:

- explore the value of trust and trustworthiness and recognise the importance of trust in the practitioner–service user relationship;

- define the origins of a duty of confidentiality and discuss the justifications for such a duty;

- examine the possible exceptions to the obligation of confidentiality;

- explore the value of honesty and truth-telling in the context of health and care;

- reflect on care strategies that promote trust and trustworthiness in practice.

INTRODUCTION

Trust and trustworthiness are among the values that seemed to lose prominence in health care ethics with the rise in emphasis placed on respect for autonomy, yet they are fundamental to health and care practice. Respect for autonomy has emerged as a primary guiding principle, with the notion of trust becoming associated with more paternalistic approaches to care. The suggestion is that placing full trust in the practitioner to do what is right and act in our best interests undermines the self-determination and control in decision-making that autonomy demands. However, trust must still be at the heart of the care relationship. It is difficult, if not impossible, to form a good therapeutic relationship without an element of trust between the individuals involved. Service users and patients need to be confident that they can trust the practitioners delivering their care to be concerned for their well-being and to act in their best interests. We seek guidance, support and care when we have health or social care needs and expect those caring for us when we are ill or vulnerable to be knowledgeable and skilled in their particular area of practice, at whatever level. However, this inevitably means that the relationship between the practitioner and those receiving care is often an unequal one, where the practitioner can be seen to hold at least some position of power over the service user or patient simply because of their role and expertise. Much work has been done in recent years to shift this balance of power and to enable patients and service users to have a voice and retain control in decision-making at individual, community, service and policy levels. This work includes increased service user involvement, participation and partnership working, and citizen and self-advocacy services. Yet trust is still an essential component. You have already seen that to be autonomous requires a number of qualities such as adequate knowledge and information and skills in critical reflection and decision making that may need to be fostered and supported through the therapeutic relationship. Thus, service users, patients and carers must still have confidence in, and be able to trust and rely on, the practitioner not only to provide relevant guidance and support but also to intervene and act appropriately with our interests in mind when required.

Experiencing trust in our daily lives

We place our trust in others every day of our lives and trust people to do what they say they will do, to play by the rules and to behave reasonably (O'Neill, 2002b). If we didn't, and couldn't, living in society would be impossible. Being able to trust makes our social life easier and worthwhile and enables us to fulfil activities that we could not achieve on our own. We trust our friends to keep secrets, the person to whom we lend money to return it, other drivers to drive carefully, nurseries to care for our children, colleagues to do what they say. Relying on one another to behave and respond in predictable ways is particularly valuable for human beings and for society as a whole.

Describing trust

'Trust' is a word used in everyday language, although a common understanding is harder to establish and it can be viewed from a number of perspectives. A standard account of trust presumes that trust depends on information and experience. It would be rare to trust people implicitly and completely. I might trust a qualified electrician to rewire my home but not to look after my child. When we trust another it is often related to a specific role or activity. However, to gain and be deserving of trust, practitioners are not only expected to be competent to do what we trust them to do but also show that they are committed to doing it, i.e. that they are trustworthy.

Trust in health and social care services

Putting your trust in another inevitably leads to an expectation that others will be both reliable and dependable, although trusting always involves an element of risk and there are no guarantees that the person or institution will live up to the expectations of the individual who has placed their trust in them. Trust in the health and social care professions has taken some significant knocks over more recent years and the centrality of trust has been threatened, perhaps even eroded, by the increase in highly publicised malpractice and misconduct cases such as that of the nurse Beverly Allitt, the GP Harold Shipman, the Kennedy Report into the problems in paediatric heart surgery at the Bristol Royal Infirmary, and the failings of the multidisciplinary team in the Victoria Climbié/Laming inquiry. While it cannot be denied that serious and inexcusable harm and suffering occurred in each of these, and similar, cases, it is important to remember that such behaviour is not reflective of the behaviour of the vast majority of practitioners. Professional bodies and sector skills councils continue to work to promote trust in practitioners through rules, standards, competency frameworks, policies and guidelines for practice. The aim to maintain trust where it already exists or to restore trust where it is threatened or diminished, and the value of trustworthiness, is reinforced and espoused in many codes of practice. Thus the importance of maintaining, justifying and enhancing the trust placed by individuals in health and care practitioners is taken seriously, whether they are professionally registered or working towards professional registration.

Although professionalism and professional codes, regulation and guidance are essential components in health and social care, not all practitioners belong to registered professions or fall under the regulation of these codes. However, any care relationship is a privileged one; practitioners or individuals in their care rarely have any real choice in whom they form a relationship with. They may have little or nothing in common with each other and yet the carer assumes a role in, and has access to, the most personal and intimate aspects of the service user or patient's lives. Thus trust is fundamental to the individual's confidence in the practitioner and, if trust breaks down at this level, it can have detrimental effects both for the patient or service user and for the service as a whole. Hence, the importance of being reliable, dependable and trustworthy applies equally to those in professionally regulated and those in unregulated assistant or support worker roles in health and social care.

Confidentiality and truth-telling

With the increasing emphasis on working in partnership with patients and service users to provide optimum care, building a relationship of mutual respect and trust is fundamental and inevitably everyone seeking advice, support or care will place an element of trust in practitioners. In particular, working in collaboration with patients, service users, carers and other members of the interprofessional team inevitably requires communication, consultation and the disclosure and sharing of information. This aspect of care gives rise to two specific duties related to the value of trust and trustworthiness – those of confidentiality and truth-telling. Having to discuss personal and sometimes difficult, intimate and otherwise private information with relative strangers calls for a degree of trust and confidence that the practitioners involved will respect the individual's privacy and confidentiality. Equally, patients and service users will expect practitioners to be truthful and honest when responding to questions and requests for information that will inform their decision-making, including the consent process. This chapter explores the value of trust and trustworthiness in health and social care and aims to assist you to reflect on your development as a trustworthy practitioner, paying particular attention to the notions of confidentiality and truthfulness.

WHAT ARE TRUST AND TRUSTWORTHINESS?

Each of us and every profession and every institution needs trust. We need it because we have to be able to rely on others acting as they say that they will, and because we need others to accept that we will act as we say we will. The sociologist Niklas Luhman was right that 'A complete absence of trust would prevent [one] even getting up in the morning'.

(O'Neill, 2002b, p.1)

And when we place trust we don't simply assume that others are reliable and predictable, as we assume that the sun rises reliably, and the milk goes off predictably. When we trust we know – at least when we are no longer small children – that we could be disappointed. Sometimes we place trust in spite of past disappointment, or without much evidence of reliability. To withdraw trust after a single lapse, as if we were rejecting a scientific theory in the face of decisive evidence, would often seem suspicious, even paranoid. All trust risks disappointment. The risk of disappointment, even of betrayal, cannot be written out of our lives. Samuel Johnson put it this way: 'It is happier to be sometimes cheated than not to trust'. Trust is needed not because everything is wholly predictable, or wholly guaranteed, but on the contrary because life has to be led without guarantees.

(O'Neill, 2002c, p.1)

Trust is an important concept in all of the human services and caring disciplines but, although trust is an everyday concept, it may be defined and utilised in a number of ways. Trust can be used to describe the foundation and nature of therapeutic relationships, as a personal attribute or as a quality of interprofessional relationships. It can also be seen as a need or as a duty or obligation of one person or persons to another, and we may place trust in individuals, groups, institutions or societies. Trust is an attitude we have towards other people who we hope will be trustworthy, whereas trustworthiness is a property or characteristic of individuals that can be described in moral terms and as a virtue.

Reflection

Think about a situation where you have placed your trust in another. This could be related to, for example, a personal friendship or someone who provides a particular service, e.g. a teacher, a plumber or a health care practitioner.

1. What was the nature of the trust you placed in them?

2. What were the key components that you felt enabled you to place your trust in them? Why did you trust this person?

3. Did you have any doubts about their trustworthiness? If so, why did you have doubts and what were they?

What you may have identified is a number of qualities of the individual, such as being reliable, being expert, having specific knowledge and skills, being competent or something about your relationship with them such as, for example, having confidence in them or being able to depend on them, even if they are relative strangers. All of these qualities are connected with the notion of trust and in being trustworthy, i.e. that you deem them worthy of your trust. Another key aspect of trust that you could have identified is that you had confidence in trusting the person because they occupied a role that is recognised and certified by associations or professional bodies who define the competence or standards of their members, usually as a result of some specific training and education. Even something as simple as taking a taxi requires an element of trust; we can check that the driver is a registered cab driver, which (hopefully) provides the assurance that he is qualified to drive. However, we have to trust that he will then drive safely, that his taxi is roadworthy and that the driver knows where he is going. We may even trust that he will take the quickest (and therefore cheapest) route.

Trust and relationships

Trust, as identified by McLeod (2006, p.1), 'is both important and dangerous'. It is important in the sense that it supports the forming of relationships with others and enables us to depend on others for such things as friendship, advice and help. Trust involves a relationship that is based on uncertain knowledge about the likely action of another and you depend on them for a beneficial outcome. It is a relationship where we rely on others to do what they say or what we expect, even if we know there is no other imperative, like a law or code, compelling them to do so. When we place our trust in others we are relying on them to take care of something that we care about, which may be something tangible, like trusting a friend to return money I have lent him, or less tangible, such as when I trust a stranger to be honest when I ask him the time or when I trust a practitioner to preserve my self-respect or well-being.

Trust exists in relationships where there are no absolute guarantees that a person has to act or behave in a certain way; if we could guarantee everyone's behaviour all of the time then the notion of trust would be redundant. For example, you expect that a car driver will slow down at a pedestrian crossing when the lights change to amber and will stop when the light is red. In this case, the law expects this too and provides a legal imperative on the driver. However, you also have to trust that the individual will observe the law and will stop at the red light – there is no absolute guarantee. Thus, trust is also 'dangerous' in that it involves an element of risk. The risk is that either or both sides may let each other down, that you may lose what you have entrusted to another to protect or that people will act in ways that harm rather than benefit the trusting individual. For this reason, trust and relationships based in trust can also be misplaced and easily and irreparably damaged.

In trusting others we place ourselves in a vulnerable position and we base our trust on the expectation that others will not take advantage of or exploit our vulnerability for their own self-interest and benefit, or for some misplaced understanding of our own good. This vulnerability may be accentuated in the therapeutic relationship, particularly if patients and service users feel apprehensive and intimidated by practitioners because of their apparent position of power and authority, resulting in an imbalance of control over decision-making and disempowerment. Self-respect can be shattered by a betrayal of trust (McLeod, 2006). This can be seen in the examples in Figure 4.1. Figure 4.2 provides a summary of the conditions for trust.

500,000 older people are victims of crime
McVeigh, K. (2007) *The Guardian*, 8 November 2007 at **www.guardian.co.uk/society/ 2007/nov/08/socialcare.longtermcare** (accessed 10 November 2007)

Elderly victims of crime will be allowed to give evidence via video links from home, prosecutors said yesterday as it emerged that up to 500,000 older people a year could fall victim to abuse and neglect, bogus traders or street crime. There is a huge under-reporting of crimes against older people, due to fear, embarrassment and a lack of access to trusted people to whom they can report their worries. One study, published this year, found that only 6% of elderly victims had reported abuse to the police. The Crown Prosecution Service said it was increasingly concerned about the abuse of society's most frail and vulnerable, particularly by those in positions of trust ... The CPS said it would focus on abuse or neglect in situations of trust, involving family members, carers or paid workers, as well as on offences against older people because of their perceived vulnerability, including muggings, doorstep theft and rogue traders, and offences wholly or partly driven by hostility linked to age.

Gesture politics are no use to youths
Butler, P. (2007) *The Guardian*, 7 November 2007 at **www.guardian.co.uk/society/ 2007/nov/07/guardiansocietysupplement.youngpeople** (accessed 10 November 2007)

What do young people want from politicians? Not lip service, media-friendly gestures, or empty promises. Trust in the political class is not high among those routinely caricatured and denigrated by ministers as 'hoodies'. So when Gordon Brown promises to spend millions to makeover England's patchy leisure facilities for teen-agers, he'd better be serious. Whatever his swing-voter focus groups might say, this has to be much more than a short-term political 'solution' to the 'youth problem'.

Carer stole £15k from old couple
BBC NEWS (2007) *BBC News On-Line*, 14 Sept 2007 at **http://news.bbc.co.uk/go/pr/ fr/-/1/hi/wales/6995693.stm** (accessed 12 November 2007)

A carer who stole £15,000 from an elderly couple's bank account after discovering their card details and pin numbers, has been jailed for 16 months.
Marian Lloyd-Davies, 43, of Bangor, Gwynedd, was branded "wicked and despicable" by a judge for stealing from the couple she was caring for. ... One of her victims suffered from Alzheimer's disease, the court heard ... the judge, Mr Recorder Phillip Heywood refused [the] request for a suspended prison sentence. As he jailed Lloyd Davies for 16 months he told her: 'You were in a position of trust. You had access to their home and you abused that trust.'

Figure 4.1 Examples of the betrayal of trust

A summary of the conditions for trust

One's attitude is conducive to trust of another if there is:

- an acceptance of some level of risk or vulnerability (regarding whether they can be trusted to do what they are depended upon to do);
- an acceptance of the risk of being let down or betrayed (which is more than just being disappointed – for example, you can rely on an alarm clock and if it breaks you are disappointed but not betrayed);
- an inclination to expect the best of the other person (at least in the areas in which you trust the person);
- optimism, not pessimism or suspicion about the person to be trusted (but optimism and lack of suspicion can make one more open to harm);
- a belief or optimism that the person is competent (in certain respects);
- a belief or optimism that the person is committed to do what they are trusted to do;
- a belief or optimism that, in general, the trusted person has a certain kind of motive for acting (controversial because it is unclear as to what motive we expect from people we trust);
- some expectation of shared moral values or norms and a moral disposition to be trustworthy; trustworthiness as a virtue.

Figure 4.2 A summary of the conditions for trust (adapted from McLeod, 2006, pp.3–8).

Types of trust

A distinction can be made between knowledge-based trust, trust in institutions and moralistic trust (Uslaner, 2001).

Knowledge-based trust

A standard account of trust is that of knowledge-based trust, which depends on information and experience. On this account, we trust people because of our past experiences, knowledge and expectations of how they will behave or act such as, for example, in the knowledge that they have previously kept their promises, have been honest or have not betrayed our secrets. A single encounter with another person is usually insufficient to establish your trust in that person; mutual trust develops through experience and is dependent on what we know about each other. For example, my colleague and I may trust each other to lend a small amount of money but I would not trust them to repair my car nor would they trust me to do the same for them as neither of us has sufficient knowledge of the other's expertise in these areas. Similarly, you may seek appointments with the same general practitioner (GP) because you have developed trust in their judgement based on your past experiences and knowledge of their approach to the consultation.

Trust in institutions

Trust in institutions has some similarities to knowledge-based trust and some distinctive qualities. Institutions can include government structures and systems, health care organisations, hospitals, social services and professional bodies and groups. Putting faith in institutions may involve confidence rather than trust because institutions cannot reciprocate your trust in the same way as in individual relationships. However, we do make judgements about our trust in institutions according to our knowledge and experience. It is this trust in institutions that becomes threatened by reports of untrustworthy actions, malpractice and misconduct by politicians, health and social care professionals, schools, exam boards, hospitals, etc. and the media presents a picture of our increasing mistrust. In response we hear claims of increased governance, regulation, standards, transparency and accountability in attempts to regain or reinforce our trust in these institutions (O'Neill, 2002b). Professional regulation and professional codes of practice are one significant measure used to define the responsibility and accountability of professional groups with a view to justifying public confidence and trust in the health and care professions.

Research activity

Find at least three different codes of practice or codes of conduct relevant to your practice setting. These may be related to the professional groups or roles within the multidisciplinary or interprofessional team in which you work such as, for example, doctors, nurses, midwives, social workers, social carers, occupational therapists, radiographers, counsellors, psychotherapists, psychologists.

Trust is hard to define and apply to a whole group or institution; it may be easier from our knowledge and experience to say that we trust some nurses but not others, that we trust a doctor to treat one condition but not another. However, service users and patients rarely get to choose the practitioner who will provide their care; instead they place their trust in another because they are members of a profession or an institution. Being regulated and observant of a code of conduct goes a significant way to providing reassurance in the professional group if we are confident that their fear of detection and punishment by their professional body is sufficient to dissuade them from breaching the code (and from causing us any consequent harm). However, this is insufficient on its own to justify and prove the trustworthiness of individual practitioners. Although a professional is presumed to seek to fulfil policies, ethical codes, the law and their previous promises, unquestioning trust in members of a professional group can be misplaced. It has been the uncritical acceptance that 'doctor always knows best' that has led to criticisms of paternalism in situations where professional dominance has impinged on the autonomy of patients or, at worst, has provided opportunities for members of professions to abuse their professional privilege, resulting in harm of those in their care. Also, a significant proportion of the health and social care team are not regulated by a professional body or bound by any specific code of conduct and yet they are just as (or more) likely to be involved in the intimate and personal aspects of an individual's care. There must be other reasons for placing trust in practitioners that goes beyond the membership of a profession.

Personal and professional trust

De Raeve (2002) debates the distinctions between personal and professional trust in the practitioner–patient relationship and this has a bearing on the discussion of the importance of trust placed in professions and non-professions. De Raeve (2002) claims that there are distinctions between those people with whom you have a personal relationship, for example, a partner or close friend, those who are members of a trade or provide a service and those who are 'professionals'. She makes the distinction between non-professional and professional work as being that between those occupations that require someone to be well-skilled and know the facts and rules of the trade and those professional occupations where judgement is also required and where rules can only operate as guidelines. De Raeve takes this distinction further in establishing that it is the complexity, the moral nature and implications of professional judgements that make the difference between the trust you might place in a tradesperson compared with the trust you place in a health professional. For example, if a plumber is careless, he would be doing bad work on my house, not on me. Although I may experience the consequences of his actions, his disregard for my interests is not the same as that of a doctor's or nurse's carelessness that may result in a direct harm to me, which is morally reprehensible, regardless of the lack of intent (de Raeve, 2002, p.154). What is also important here is that the professional is held to account for their actions and takes responsibility for ensuring that I can rely on them.

Although de Raeve creates this distinction between non-professional and professional groups, the same obligations of trust are placed on other carers and practitioners who are not members of a regulated profession but are seen as belonging to the same service (such as the NHS or social services) or who form a significant part of the multidisciplinary team. These practitioners also carry significant responsibility to conduct themselves and act in ways that do not undermine public trust and confidence (and the GSCC Code of Practice for Social Care Workers (2002) applies equally to those in regulated and registered professions and those in support, assistant and associate practitioner roles). What also matters in the therapeutic relationship is the notion of moralistic trust or trustworthiness.

Moral responsibility and trustworthiness

We have already seen that trust in others may stem from our knowledge and experience and it may also stem from their membership or belonging to institutions such as professional groups or care sectors and services. To justify trust, practitioners must also take responsibility for their role, the way in which their behaviour will influence and impact on individuals' lives, and they must ensure that they can be relied upon in helping individuals to make their own decisions about their health and welfare (or even make these decisions on their behalf when necessary). In placing their trust, service users inevitably have to allow practitioners some discretion to fulfil their responsibilities; they have to rely, to some degree, on the expertise and knowledge of the practitioner. However, this does not give practitioners total freedom to do as they please and it is because of the risk associated with relying on others for care and support that trustworthiness is so important. Moralistic trust is a moral commandment to treat people as if they were trustworthy (Uslaner, 2001). Thus, what is also fundamental to trustworthy behaviour is a strong sense and understanding of your moral values in relating to others, sensitivity and appreciation of their value positions and taking moral responsibility for your own judgements and actions in your everyday practice. Practitioners must be motivated to act in a trustworthy manner if they are to justify the trust placed in them (Smith, 2005, p.302).

Discussion activity

1. Make a list of the characteristics you believe are essential to being trustworthy.

2. Ask three colleagues to list what they consider to be the key characteristics. Ideally ask people who hold different roles and responsibilities within the multidisciplinary team such as, for example, a nurse, a social worker, a doctor, a counsellor, a therapist, a teacher.

3. Compare and contrast your lists and discuss the similarities and differences with your colleagues.

4. Try to think of reasons for the similarities and differences.

Trustworthiness is often referred to as a virtue (a quality of character that is morally good) and means being worthy of others' trust. That is, that you will have a strong sense that morally right behaviour is important in your dealings with others. Being morally trustworthy also assumes that you will act according to appropriate moral norms and will have a good will or motive to your actions. Annette Baier (1986) connected this with a caring disposition. Moral norms or values associated with being trustworthy include:

- demonstrating respect for others;
- honesty;
- integrity;
- openness;
- responsiveness;
- caring for their well-being and having concern for their welfare;
- being fair;
- keeping promises and keeping confidences.

Trustworthiness also requires other interpersonal behaviours such as understanding service users' individual experiences, communicating clearly and completely, and building partnerships (Thom and Campbell, 1997). People also expect that the trustworthy practitioner will respond in a moral way to their trusting behaviour and not betray their trust, i.e. that you will not take advantage of their vulnerability. Trusting a practitioner incorporates an expectation of a beneficial response even though they could do harm (Smith, 2005, p.302).

Practitioners cannot simply assume that patients and service users will place trust in them solely because of the role they hold, be they nurse, doctor, social worker, care assistant, etc. Demonstrating their knowledge and competence alone is not enough for the development and mainte-nance of the trust that is so essential to the therapeutic relationship (Hupcey and Miller, 2006). Confidence in the organisation to provide reliable and competent practitioners provides a threshold of safe care from which trust can emerge but, although this is sufficient to be a reliable practitioner, trustworthiness must grow from this as you build the care relationship with the patient or service user. Given that different service users' perceptions of trustworthiness will vary, it is essential that care is individualised. The service user's trust will generally be well founded when the person they entrust is dependable, reliable and cred-ible and willing to stand by their own moral standards, i.e. has moral integrity. Their degree of trust may be seen in their belief in your honesty, openness, reliability, sincerity, benevolence, kindness, compassion, self-lessness and competence. However, this is a tall order for any practitioner. Trust with service users can take a long time to establish but can be destroyed in an instant through carelessness or a thoughtless act. It is therefore essential that you work hard to establish and maintain the trust of those in your care by practising with moral sensitivity, care, compassion and respect. Two key areas of practice which are essential in establishing and maintaining trust in the care relationship are the principles related to confidentiality and truth-telling.

CONFIDENTIALITY AND TRUTH-TELLING

The principles of confidentiality and truth-telling are seen as fundamental characteristics of the trust placed in therapeutic relationships in health and social care. However, they may also come into conflict with other important obligations like, for example, to do no harm, to act in a person's best interests or when balancing the interests of the individual in your care against those of others.

Introduction to the principle of confidentiality

The duty to maintain patient or service user confidentiality is fundamental to health and social care and is enshrined in the law, ethics and in professional codes of practice and conduct. Practitioners have access to, and are entrusted with, wide-ranging information about their patients and service users and never has confidentiality been as important as in our increasing technological and 'information age'. Confidentiality has traditionally been associated with the one-to-one relationship between service users and practitioners. However, with the introduction of single assessment processes and electronic records, different groups of practitioners will have varying levels of access to information about the patient or service user, extending the opportunities for breach of confidentiality. With the phasing in of the NHS Care Records Service from 2007, NHS organisations will increasingly keep care records on networked computers, which will allow staff quicker access to information across organisational boundaries. Similar developments and their associated challenges exist for social care. As care packages and the care team become more varied, encompassing new interprofessional roles and crossing multidisciplinary boundaries, the debate surrounding the nature and extent to which information should be shared and with whom is becoming increasingly complex. This shift from single practitioner–service user relationships to one of health and social care services–service user relationships means there is increasing need for trusted and trustworthy systems to keep information private (what the British Medical Association refer to as an 'information governance model' (BMA, 2005)) as well as being able to have continued confidence in individual practitioners not to breach confidences without good reason.

Confidentiality is protected in common law, in professional codes and standards and in contractual obligations to employers such that any unjustified breach of confidentiality can result in both a legal action of negligence or the accusation of professional misconduct, as well as disciplinary proceedings related to breach of contracts of employment. However, it is recognised that any duty of confidentiality cannot be absolute and careful consideration has to be given to the legal and moral limits on any duty of confidentiality.

Reflection

Defining confidentiality

1. Think about the last time you told someone something 'in confidence'. Was there anything special or different about the information and, if so, in what ways?

2. Why did you disclose this information and what did you expect of the other person/s with regard to this information?

3. How did you convey your expectations with regard to how the other person would treat the information?

4. Are you confident that the person did not disclose the information to anyone else? How would you feel if they had?

Defining confidentiality

Use of the term 'confidentiality' or telling someone something 'in confidence' generally implies an element of trust to keep secret that which is disclosed to a person or persons and usually pertains to private and personal information. If you think back to the discussion about trust, to trust another always involves an element of risk so, in sharing information in confidence, you may well also attempt to protect yourself from risk by invoking a promise from the person you have confided in. How often have you said, 'I'll tell you this but you must promise not to tell anyone'? However, your belief in their trustworthiness is still important because you still have to trust that the person will also keep their promises.

Believing in the notion of confidentiality in itself therefore provides you with the confidence to share specific information that you would otherwise protect from the intrusion of others. In health and social care, individuals place significant trust in practitioners that the otherwise private and personal information that they share with you will be protected and they entrust this to you with the intent that it will be used for their benefit such as, for example, to secure a diagnosis or to receive the appropriate care, support or advice.

Why is confidentiality important in health and social care?

Every day health and care workers are party to confidential information, usually given openly and willingly or acquired through the assessment process and care relationship. It would be near impossible to carry out accurate, effective and appropriate care without a certain amount of personal and private information about the service user and they generally give it with the expectation that it will be used to their benefit. You are therefore in a privileged position to receive and be entrusted with this private information and it should be obvious from the earlier discussion in Chapter 2 that a duty of confidentiality is required from the value of respect for the person, their privacy and their autonomy as well as from the value of trust and being trustworthy. Consider the question, 'what information is subject to a duty of confidentiality?'

Confidential information

Confidential information is any information that is given to you in confidence, that is not freely available through normal social discourse and that is given when one individual trusts another. You have to be careful here because what you would disclose to others in normal conversation may not be the same standard as that set by the service user. Certainly, any personal information related to their physical, mental and emotional health and well-being should be treated as confidential. In English law, a duty of confidentiality will usually be recognised (Mason *et al.*, 2005) if:

- information is of a private or intimate nature;
- information is given to another in a situation where there is an obligation not to disclose it, i.e. a relationship of trust;
- protection of confidentiality is in the public interest or where the service user would suffer if the information was revealed;
- a breach of confidentiality would involve an unauthorised disclosure or use of the information.

The fact that individuals believe and trust that information passed to the practitioner will be kept a secret, and therefore given with confidence, is fundamental to the therapeutic care relationship. Service users and patients must believe that they can talk honestly and frankly without fear of exposure, otherwise they may withhold information important not only to their health but possibly to the well-being of others. Jones

(2003) found that patients clearly value confidentiality, see it as important to the medical consultation, and recognise that disclosure of information to others without their consent might deter patients from seeking treatment. However, according to British Medical Association (BMA, 2005) research, service users' views regarding their expectations of confidentiality are varied; they generally appear to want their information kept securely (not perhaps surprising, particularly as we hear more and more about identity theft and fraudulent activity) but also want relevant information to be readily available and shared with those that need it in order to deliver the best care. Some individuals also believe that the benefits of maintaining confidentiality could be outweighed by disclosure if it were for the prevention of harm and protection of third parties (Jones, 2003). They become more concerned regarding access to information as the request or need moves further away from those directly involved in delivering care, with particular worries associated with access by employers, insurers, social workers and benefit agencies (BMA, 2005, p.6). For example, if service users receiving care for mental illness, drug addiction or HIV infection believed that employers might have access to their medical records, this would prove a big disincentive to them seeking advice, health care and support. There has also been a shift in emphasis to place obligations on institutions such as the NHS and other care services to take steps to ensure that confidential information is subject to data protection, which recognises the increased risk of breaches of confidence and invasion of privacy through the storage and use of computerised service user records.

Research activity

1. Locate the most recent guidance on confidentiality on the Department of Health website. At the time of publication, this is the Department of Health NHS Code of Practice for Confidentiality (DoH, 2003b) located at **www.dh.gov.uk/en/Policyand guidance/Informationpolicy/Patientconfidentialityandcaldicott guardians/DH_4100550** (accessed 16 November 2007).

This Code (p.3):
- introduces the concept of confidentiality;
- describes what a confidential service should look like;
- provides a high level description of the main legal requirements;
- recommends a generic decision support tool for sharing/disclosing information;
- lists examples of particular information disclosure scenarios.

> 2. Find the 'Confidentiality model' in this code that sets out four main requirements that must be met to provide a confidential service. What are these requirements?
>
> 3. Make some summary notes explaining each of these requirements.
>
> 4. Although this relates to National Health Service organisations and practitioners, the general principles are also transferable to a range of settings and organisations in health and social care. Can you identify evidence of these requirements being met in your care setting? Write down some examples.

The Department of Health *NHS Code of Practice for Confidentiality* (DoH, 2003b), published in response to the increased complexity of maintaining confidentiality, is a guide to required practice. Along with a number of guiding principles, it requires health and social care organisations to appoint 'Caldicott Guardians' to ensure the protection of confidential information throughout the organisation. The requirement for a Caldicott Guardian was later rolled out to social care organisations and there are now at least 750 registered Caldicott Guardians working within the NHS, social care and other health-related organisations. There are also laws to protect and control data sharing, including the Data Protection Act 1998 and Access to Medical Reports Act 1988. These Acts also give service users rights to know what information has been recorded about them, which is also important to their trust in care services (see Dimond, 2004, Chapter 8, 'Data protection: confidentiality and access' for a more detailed exploration of the law associated with access to medical records and data protection).

Although the systems, structures and laws to prevent inappropriate storage and use of service user data are extremely important in today's health and social care, what we are more concerned with here are your duties and obligations related to confidentiality that arise from the value of trust and respect for persons in the one-to-one relationships of caring.

What are the origins of any duty to respect confidences?

Confidentiality is one of the most deeply respected moral commitments in health care (Gillon, 1986). It is enshrined in many codes of practice and dates back to Hippocrates and the Hippocratic Oath (originally sworn by doctors on entering the medical profession) that stated:

> Whatever, in connection with my professional practice, or not in connection with it, I see or hear, in the life of men, which ought not

to be spoken of abroad, I will not divulge, as reckoning that all such should be kept secret.

More recently, the modern version of the oath, the Declaration of Geneva (2006), extended this expectation of confidentiality to individuals even after their death, stating, 'I will respect the secrets which are confided in me, even after the patient has died'. Although much is written about medical confidentiality, by inference, and arising from their own professional codes of conduct and legal and moral principles, all other health and care practitioners are required to respect a duty of confidentiality.

Research activity

1. Go back to the codes of practice or codes of conduct relevant to your practice setting that you identified in the earlier section on trust. Compare and contrast the expectations regarding confidentiality in the codes for different professional or practitioner groups (for example those for doctors, nurses, midwives, social workers, social carers, occupational therapists, radiographers, counsellors, psychotherapists, psychologists).

2. Summarise the similarities and differences between the codes you have reviewed and consider the implications for your practice.

Codes of practice obviously place a significant duty on individual practitioners in health and social care to preserve confidentiality and not to reveal patient or service user information that is otherwise private and personal, although most codes suggest there may be some exceptions to this rule. Different organisations and professional groups may vary in their policies and practices regarding confidentiality and it may be that access to service user records or particular aspects of their information is limited to specific members of the health or social care team. However, everybody in a care relationship will be privy to some personal and potentially intimate information about the service user, so the duty of confidentiality is not restricted to those in professional roles. Confidentiality is everybody's business. The reasons, aside from professional codes, why health and care workers have a duty to uphold confidentiality (Dimond, 2004) arise from:

- a duty of care owed to those with whom you have a therapeutic relationship (this originates from the common law of tort and negligence);
- the implied duty under a contract of employment;

- duties created by statutes, especially the Data Protection Act 1998 and Article 8 'Right to respect for private and family life' of the Human Rights Act 1998;
- a duty to keep information passed on in confidence confidential even when there is no pre-existing relationship or legally enforceable contract between parties, i.e. based on equity.

There is also a moral duty arising from the value of respect for persons and respect for privacy as a citizen, and from the duty to promote their welfare through the development of a trusting relationship.

THE MORAL VALUE OF MAINTAINING CONFIDENTIALITY

A moral duty of confidentiality exists if the following necessary conditions are met (Gillon, 1985):

- One person must disclose to another information that they regard as secret.
- The other person must (implicitly or explicitly) undertake not to reveal the first person's secrets.

The obligation to keep secrets arises from the value placed on respect for persons and their privacy, respect for their autonomy and the fact that harm may follow if the secret is revealed. We have already discussed the importance of people being able to have control over their own lives and make their own choices and this value extends to decisions about if, when and with whom their personal information should be shared. You have also seen that privacy is an essential component of maintaining dignity. Thus, if you are told a 'secret', it is usually knowledge that you have an obligation to conceal. According to Garrett *et al.* (2001, pp.118–9) the types of obligatory secrets are:

1. the natural secret;
2. the promised secret;
3. the professional secret.

The natural secret

The natural secret is so named because the information involved is, by its very nature, potentially harmful if revealed – for example, private and intimate information. If the obligation to avoid harm is universal, i.e. owed by everyone and not just by those in professional or contractual relationships, then even the lay person is obliged to keep such a secret, for example, that a friend has had a positive HIV test. The obligation exists regardless of how the information was obtained. In this instance, even a person's name can be confidential if revealing it may cause them some embarrassment or harm. However, there may still be exceptions where the benefits of keeping such secrets are outweighed by the benefits of disclosure. For example, imagine a thief who you caught red-handed saying, 'ssh, don't tell the police, it's a secret!'

The promised secret

The promised secret is knowledge that we have promised to conceal. Generally, the promise exists because the information is also a natural secret. However, the particular harm associated with revealing a promised secret arises not only from the sensitivity of the information but also from the harmful effects of breaking promises. Service users may well assume that practitioners, simply through their relationship of providing care, have made an implied promise to keep their secrets, even when no express promise has been made. This is why it is particularly important to state that you cannot promise to always keep their information secret if there are circumstances where there may be some overriding duty to disclose, such as cases where it may place the service user at risk of significant harm if the information is not disclosed or where the law requires disclosure of information (we consider possible exceptions to a duty of confidentiality in the next section). However, we generally depend on people in our social life to keep promises and most of us would be wary of the person we cannot trust to keep a promise, so exceptions have to be minimised. That said, there are obviously limits to the extent of our promise-keeping depending on the balance of harms and benefits. For example, a person would be justified in revealing the intention of a friend to kill even if they have sworn to keep it secret.

The professional secret

The professional secret is knowledge that is obtained in a professional relationship that, if revealed, will harm not only the service user but may also do serious harm to the profession and to the society that depends on that profession for important services. The duty to protect professional secrets is enshrined in the law or the code of practice but is also justified through the moral value of trust. The importance of the professional secret can be best seen by contemplating the consequences of a loss of trust in the practitioner or professional group or service. If service users cannot trust you to keep their secrets, they may feel betrayed and may be reluctant to disclose important information essential to their care or it may prevent them seeking further support or treatment (this links back to the notion of knowledge-based trust where people validate their trust in you through their experiences and trust is dependent on what they know about you). This could result in care being inappropriate because it is based on inadequate or incomplete facts. Also, if a particular service user reveals to others that their confidence has been breached, this may have a knock-on effect for the overall confidence in that service by other members of the public (see also the notion of trust in institutions discussed earlier in this chapter), ultimately putting the health and well-being of others potentially at risk. Without trust and respect of confidences the fabric of society would be threatened, and people's health, welfare and overall good may be affected if trust in health and care practitioners were to deteriorate. For example, if people cannot rely on confidences being respected they are less likely to seek medical help in the case of sexually transmitted infections. In this case, it is in the interests of the individual and society that the patient can ask for advice in confidence.

Thus there are very good legal, professional and moral reasons for valuing confidentiality and respecting a duty of confidentiality. However, you may already be raising questions in your own mind as to whether or not you should always maintain confidentiality or whether there may sometimes be exceptions to this rule.

IS THE DUTY OF CONFIDENTIALITY AN ABSOLUTE DUTY?

In order to care in the most appropriate manner for patients and service users, and given that health and social care involves interprofessional, multidisciplinary and multi-agency approaches, it would be impossible for confidentiality to be an absolute principle. Nevertheless, any breaches of confidentiality should be exceptional and the duty of confidentiality should be a *prima facie* obligation (i.e. it must be maintained unless it conflicts on a particular occasion with an equal or stronger obligation). Therefore, the difficulty is not in identifying the value of respect for confidentiality but in explaining or defining any exceptions to such a duty.

Imaginative exercise

Think about the incident of the thief that you catch red-handed who says 'ssh, don't tell the police, it's a secret!' It would seem relatively uncontroversial to breach their confidence and report them to the police.

Now imagine that, instead, you come across this person while working in Accident and Emergency. They reveal to you that their injuries relate to a theft they have just committed but state, 'please keep this a secret, promise you won't tell the police, I needed the money to buy food for my family'.

1. Should you respect this patient's confidences in this case? Explain your answer.

2. What exceptions are there to any duty of confidentiality?

As a practitioner you voluntarily undertake a general commitment to keep secrets and there is a contractual care relationship between the patient and practitioner that would justify maintaining the patient's confidences. Certainly, if you consider the value placed on respect for persons (regardless of their actions), then your first concerns would be the treatment and care required in relation to their injury. You may feel there is something intrinsically wrong with allowing illegal activity to go unheeded because of the harm they have caused to others but there is no legal duty to report minor crime to the police and your duty to preserve the trust relationship should take priority. On the other hand, you should not purposefully obstruct the police in their investigations by, for example, giving false or misleading information and you can be required by a court to give evidence or disclose relevant information through a court order.

Exceptions to the duty of confidentiality

It is generally accepted in law, professional codes (and with moral justification) that confidentiality is a fundamental principle in health and care and there should be no use or disclosure of any service user information other than for the care of the person to whom it relates. However, there are three broad exceptions to this standard that can be morally justified and are recognised in the law and codes of practice (e.g. GSCC, 2002; NMC, 2004; BMA, 2005), as well as specific legal requirements that impose obligations to breach confidentiality. These are:

- consent;
- the best interests of the service user;
- the public interest.

Consent

If service users give their consent to the use or disclosure of information then this gives you permission to breach their confidence. This is the least controversial of the exceptions, although it does assume that the necessary conditions for consent have been satisfied – having capacity, being informed and freedom in decision-making (the same conditions needed to making autonomous choices). However, the requirement of consent also means that you must honour informed refusal of consent to disclose even if the disclosure is, on your account, in their best interests unless this can be justified from another stronger obligation.

Disclosure in the best interests of the service user

The need to share information with other members of the multidisciplinary, interprofessional or multi-agency team will inevitably be essential to deliver the best and most appropriate care packages for many service users. However, this 'need to know' exception should not be taken as giving complete freedom to practitioners to permit unconsidered and uncontrolled disclosure purely on the basis of another's status as a care professional or simply because they work within a service. What is potentially harming to the trust relationship between the service user and practitioner is their loss of control over their personal information. Thus, the need for information sharing among practitioners should be based in a genuine need related to that person's care and not simply disclosed on the basis of another's curiosity.

Case study

(adapted from an *Every Child Matters* Integrated Working Exemplar at **www.everychildmatters.gov.uk/_files/65C2FB97D8CBB50E8D7755 899D529E4D.pdf** (accessed 14 November 2007)

Jane suspects that she may be pregnant. She is 15 years old. Jane visits the drop-in health centre on her school site, which is provided as part of extended school services. She has her pregnancy confirmed through access to free pregnancy testing. She thinks that she is about 12 weeks pregnant. Jane is offered confidential and impartial advice from a nurse, Femi, who is attached to the centre. Jane has been reluctant to tell her parents as she is worried about their reaction. As Jane is only 15, Femi is concerned for Jane's welfare and the circumstances surrounding her pregnancy. She asks Jane about the father, reminding her that any information she gives will be regarded as confidential and will not be shared, unless not to do so would place her at risk of significant harm. Jane refuses to name the father but tells Femi that he is in Year 11, is 16 years old and was her boyfriend until they split up about a month ago.

1. Who, if anyone, needs to know that Jane is pregnant?

2. If you were Femi, what would you do next? Does she have any responsibilities that override her duty of confidentiality?

3. Now go to the worked exemplars on the *Every Child Matters* website, and follow links to the section for the 'Integrated working exemplar: teenage sexual health and pregnancy'. See how this case study continues.

Check out your answers against the Common Core of Skills and Knowledge for the Children's Workforce (Department for Education and Skills (DfES), 2005), particularly the core statements related to Effective Communication with Children, Young People and Families and Safeguarding and Promoting the Welfare of the Child).

In this case, the duty to respect confidentiality applies as much to Jane as it does to any other person over the age of 18, providing you were confident that she had sufficient maturity to form relationships of trust and understand what it means to keep promises and to trust another with a secret. Thus, duties of confidentiality and competence need not necessarily be dependent on each other, although they would be for the very young child. In addition, this duty of confidentiality would be subject to the same exceptions as those that could be applied to an adult. If a child is deemed 'Gillick competent' then disclosure without their consent would normally be unlawful (see Hendrick, 2004, pp.209–15 for a discussion of competence and consent). If you work with children and young people you should be aware of the importance of child protection law, particularly the Children Act 1989, and should be conversant with, and practise at all times, in accordance with national and local policies and guidelines for safeguarding and protecting children and young people. The Mental Capacity Act 2005 generally applies to people who are aged 16 or older. However, Chapter 12 of the Mental Capacity Act 2005 Code of Practice (Department for Constitutional Affairs, 2007) explains how the Act affects children and young people, in particular those aged 16 and 17, and you would be strongly advised to read this if you work with children and young people in this age group.

Overruling the duty of confidentiality on the basis of acting in the best interests of the service user is particularly challenging in cases where the capacity of an adult to determine for themselves what is in their best interests in a given instance is called into question. You need to think back here to the discussion about being autonomous, competence and respect for autonomy in Chapter 3. You should always start from the position of assuming someone has the capacity to make a decision for themselves unless it can be established that they lack capacity.

Throughout the *Mental Capacity Act 2005 Code of Practice* (DCA, 2007), mental capacity is defined simply as the ability to make a decision (a particular decision at the time it needs to be made), which includes decisions that affect daily life (for example, deciding when to get up or what to wear), as well as more serious or significant decisions that may have legal consequences for them or others such as, for example, deciding whether to give consent for medical treatment, buying goods or making a will (see Figure 4.3, Assessing capacity). Also, from the principle of fairness and treating everyone equally, a person's capacity must not be judged simply on the basis of their age, appearance, condition or an aspect of their behaviour.

Assessing capacity

Anyone assessing someone's capacity to make a decision for themselves should use the two-stage test of capacity included in the Mental Capacity Act 2005 (DCA, 2005, pp.44–5):

Stage 1: Does the person have an impairment of, or a disturbance in the functioning of, their mind or brain? This could include conditions associated with some forms of mental illness, dementia, significant learning disabilities, long-term effects of brain damage, physical or medical conditions that cause confusion, drowsiness or loss of consciousness and symptoms of alcohol or drug use.

Stage 2: Does the impairment or disturbance mean that the person is unable to make a specific decision when they need to?

Assessing ability to make a decision (DCA, 2007, p. 41):
- Does the person have a general understanding of what decision they need to make and why they need to make it?
- Does the person have a general understanding of the likely consequences of making, or not making, this decision?
- Is the person able to understand, retain, use and weigh up the information relevant to this decision?
- Can the person communicate their decision (by talking, using sign language or any other means)? Would the services of a professional (such as a speech and language therapist) be helpful?

Assessing capacity to make more complex or serious decisions:
- Is there a need for a more thorough assessment (perhaps by involving a doctor or other professional expert)?

Figure 4.3 Assessing capacity (adapted from the Mental Capacity Act 2005 (DCA, 2005 p.45) and the *Mental Capacity Act 2005 Code of Practice* (DCA, 2007, p.41)

Care must be taken when using judgements about mental capacity as a justification for breach of confidentiality on the basis of best interests. Think about this as you complete the next activity.

Imaginative exercise

You are the named care assistant for Tom, an 82-year-old gentleman who attends the day centre three times a week. He lives alone but has a son who calls in on him at home several times a week. Tom can be forgetful and sometimes gets confused about times of day and people's names but enjoys coming to the centre for the company of friends and joins in with all the activities. One day, he seems quieter than usual and you notice that he has some bruising on his forearms. When you sit down to talk to him, he tells you that a man has been coming to his house and has taken some money; you establish that this is probably his son. On further questioning, Tom says that his son can be a bit rough with him but implores you to keep this a secret because he loves his son and would not want him to get into any trouble, especially as he is so busy and helps him so much.

1. What would you do in these circumstances?

2. Would you be justified in breaching confidentiality in Tom's best interests?

3. Discuss this case with colleagues and compare your responses.

You would obviously need more information in a case like this before you could make a truly informed decision about whether or not you would be justified in breaching your duty of confidentiality. Tom is certainly not consenting to you sharing this information with anyone. Also, you cannot make an assumption, based on the facts here, that Tom is incompetent to make his own decisions regarding what information can be shared with others and he has already asked you to promise not to break his trust. Certainly, age on its own is not a sufficient criterion to question an adult's competence. Continuing to maintain a good care relationship based on trust, so that you can check out the facts and establish why he does not wish you to involve anyone else, may be more important at this time than disclosure. You should take all possible steps to support the person to make the decision for themselves regarding whether any action should be taken (or not). Good communication and interpersonal skills are essential in assessing capacity and in establishing other information on which you can base your decision-making. You may feel that this is outside of your role and responsibility. If so, you could consult a supervisor for advice using a hypothetical situation first before you risk breaking the service user's confidence. However, throughout this time you must be careful to monitor any changes in the situation, maintain accurate records of your observations and be prepared to act if you believe the service user is at serious risk of harm. Decisions like these will become easier as you develop your skills of professional judgement.

Disclosure in the public interest

There is also a moral, legal and professional exception to confidentiality where you can justify, in exceptional circumstances, that the rights to confidentiality are outweighed by the public interest, i.e. in order to serve a broader societal interest. Decisions to breach confidences in the public interest are complex and can only be justified when the public interest in disclosure of information outweighs the public interest in protecting confidentiality. Because the public interest in maintaining the provision of confidential health and social care services is considerable (and is fundamental to trust in these services), breaches of confidentiality in the public interest should only be considered if there are weighty justifications to overrule the practitioner's *prima facie* duty of confidentiality, and these breaches should be kept to a minimum. Justifications from the argument of the public interest include (Jackson, 2006, pp.339–55):

- preventing harm to others;
- preventing or detecting crime;
- statutory requirements.

If the risk of harm to others is used to justify disclosure, you must be confident that there is a real risk of serious harm. In cases where the individual concerned will not consent to disclosure, breaching confidentiality should only be considered if the threat posed is significant and imminent and disclosure can prevent or limit the expected harm (Jackson, 2006). The most frequently stated case in law that supports the rule of breach in the public interest is that of W *v*. Edgell.

Case study

W *v*. Edgell [1990] 1 ALL ER 835

(This case study is taken from the UK Clinical Ethics Network at **www.ethics-network.org.uk/ethical-issues/confidentiality/legal-considerations** (accessed 22 November 2007))

The patient was a prisoner in a secure hospital following convictions for killing five people and wounding several others. He made an application to a mental health tribunal to be transferred to a regional unit. An independent psychiatrist, Dr Edgell, was asked by W's legal advisers to provide a confidential expert opinion that they hoped would show that W was no longer a danger to the public. However Dr Edgell was of the opinion that in fact W was still dangerous. W's application was withdrawn. Dr Edgell, knowing that his opinion would not be included in the patient's notes, sent a copy to the medical director of the hospital and to the Home Office. The patient brought an action (against Dr Edgell) for breach of confidence.

The Court of Appeal held that the breach was justified in the public interest, on grounds of protection of the public from dangerous criminal acts. However, the Court said the risk must be 'real, immediate and serious'.

This case established that, in order to justify disclosure in the public interest, you must prove:

- there is an imminent, real and serious risk of danger to the public (and disclosure can only be justified as long as the threat persists);
- disclosure must be to a person with a legitimate interest in receiving the information, e.g. 'the responsible authorities';
- disclosure should be confined to the disclosure of information that is strictly necessary (revealing some aspects of information in the public interests does not justify disclosure of all his/her details).

Therefore, you would be justified in breaching confidentiality in cases where the disclosure would (Hendrick, 2004, p.124):

- prevent a serious risk of crime such as, for example, murder, manslaughter, gun crime, child abuse;
- prevent threats to national security;
- prevent serious risk of harm such as, for example, child abuse or neglect, spread of infectious disease, assault, serious fraud or theft;
- when required by statute.

A number of statutes (law established by a legislative body, such as Acts of Parliament) create specific exceptions to the duty of confidentiality. Some of these are listed in Figure 4.4.

It is essential that you consider very carefully the need for any possible breach of confidentiality and seek other forms of action, such as attempting to gain the consent from the service user for disclosure or finding other ways of minimising harm (to the service user themselves or the wider

The law requires or permits disclosure of confidential information under the following circumstances.

- When the requirement under the Abortion Act 1967 to provide the name and address of the woman is concerned.
- Section 60 of the Health and Social Care Act 2001 – 'enables the Secretary of State to support and regulate the use of confidential patient information in the interest of patients or the wider public good ... to ensure that patient identifiable information currently needed to support essential NHS activity can be used, without the consent that should normally be obtained, where there is no reasonably practicable alternative.'
- The Commission for Healthcare Audit and Inspection (CHAI/the Healthcare Commission) can access information under the Health and Social Care (Community Health and Standards) Act 2003.
- Control of Substances Hazardous to Health (COSHH) Regulations controlled by the Health and Safety Executive.
- Public Health (Control of Disease) Act 1984.
- National Health Service (Venereal Disease) Regulations 1974.
- Misuse of Drugs (Notification of and Supply of Addicts) Regulations 1973.
- Laws affecting all citizens that can require disclosure, e.g. Prevention of Terrorism (Temporary Provisions) Act 1989 and the Road Traffic Act 1988.
- The courts, some tribunals and persons appointed to hold inquiries have legal powers to require that information which may be relevant to matters within their jurisdiction be disclosed.
- Disclosure in criminal cases under the Criminal Procedure and Investigations Act 1996.
- Disclosure to a coroner's court. The coroners' courts have a statutory right to require the supply of information which could include personal health information.

Figure 4.4 When the law requires or permits disclosure of confidential information (taken from BMA, 2005, pp.5–6)

public interest), before you resort to breaking their confidence and potentially damaging their trust in the care relationship. You must also be careful to protect information from improper disclosure at all times and keep any service user notes securely, and not inadvertently breach your duty of confidentiality when answering phone calls or through careless and casual talk in public places. Confidentiality must also be respected when talking to relatives. They do not have an automatic right to know so, wherever possible, you should seek the permission of the service user first.

Reflection

The following are questions you could use in your reflections on this section.

1. Why do you think that confidentiality in health and social care is so important?

2. How can you ensure it is protected?

3. Why is confidentiality not an absolute duty?

4. When must you obtain the service user's permission to communicate with others about them?

5. What would you do if a service user revealed to you that they were HIV positive but refused to tell their partner or give you consent to share this information with any other practitioner?

If we value trust, then preserving the service user's right to confidentiality is one way of achieving this. However, there will be occasions when the arguments for disclosure will outweigh your duty to maintain confidentiality. What is important to minimising the loss of trust and helping to maintain the therapeutic relationship in these circumstances is that you reassure the service user that they will still be cared for and that you are honest with them about why you must breach confidentiality. Being honest and telling the truth is another fundamental component of being trustworthy.

THE VALUE OF HONESTY AND TRUTH-TELLING

Truth is an important value in our everyday lives; we do not want (or like) to be deceived and equally we find it difficult to deceive others. However, the value attributed to truth-telling is not as straightforward as it might at first appear. Even in our closest relationships, we choose what we will disclose and what will remain unsaid. This may be because we think our honesty would hurt, may be to 'keep the peace', may be because something would take too long to explain. Telling the truth relates closely to respect for the person as well as the value of trust in relationships. We started to identify the importance of being told the truth in our discussion of being autonomous and respect for autonomy, particularly when it comes down to the giving of information on which people will base their choices and decisions in health and care. However, being honest is not necessarily easy, especially when we feel the truth may hurt those receiving it. Obvious examples are where there is a poor prognosis such as, for example, with a terminal illness, cancer, Alzheimer's disease or results of genetic testing that reveal the presence of a genetic condition (such as Huntington's disease) that will occur later in life.

Reflection (adapted from Downie and Calman, 1994, p.160)

This exercise is intended to establish your attitudes towards the rights and wrongs of truth-telling with service users. Think about the following questions in relation to your practice. Do you think all or only some are morally justified? Think of examples for each and think about how you would justify your approach if called to account for your actions. Are there circumstances:

- When you would not tell the truth?
- When you would tell a lie?
- When you would not tell the whole truth?
- When you would force the truth on a person, i.e. confront them with the truth for their own good?

Why should you tell service users the truth?

The ordinary ethics of truthfulness, according to Garrett *et al.* (2001, p.112) are encompassed in two duties, namely:

- first, that you should not lie;
- second, that you should communicate with those who have a right to the truth.

Yet, these seem far too simple to explain the complex problems met in real life where truth-telling and lying can be seen to be at two ends of a continuum, with evading the truth, deception and the notion of 'little white lies' falling in between. The first statement seems to leave you free not to communicate (perhaps even to evade the question) and the second raises the question, 'who has the right to be told the truth?' Neither statement says that you must tell everyone everything you know or everything they want to know. However, we grow up believing (on the whole) that 'honesty is the best policy'.

Discussion activity

Ask colleagues what they believe about being honest and telling the truth to service users/patients.

1. Do they always tell the truth to service users/patients?

2. If not, what exceptions do they identify? How do they justify not telling the truth?

Now find out the perceptions of friends and family regarding the importance of truth-telling in health and social care.

3. Do they believe health and care practitioners always tell the truth to service users/patients? If not, why is this?

4. Do they think practitioners should always tell the truth? Why?

There are a number of justifications why, as a practitioner, you should be honest and tell service users the truth.

Respect for persons and their autonomy

Information giving is one of the necessary conditions to enable a person to be self-determining or autonomous and it is important that the information provided is honest and true (as far as we can know the truth at any particular time). If you restrict or withhold information from the service user that could otherwise inform their desires, choices and decisions, you are inevitably influencing (and possibly preventing) their opportunity to be autonomous, reducing their ability to be in control of their lives and failing to show respect for persons. Service users need information, not only to enable them to make autonomous choices, but also to inform them about their situation regardless of whether there is a choice or decision to be made. The truth will help them to plan their care, seek support and attention when needed and to make life decisions that they would not make if they were unaware of their situation or condition.

The expectation of informed consent

It follows from the information condition of being autonomous that knowing the truth is also necessary for service users to give informed consent. Giving consent in health and social care is a very real expression of the trust placed in the practitioner as consent usually involves devolving some element of responsibility for that person's health and well-being to someone else, such as a doctor, with the expectation that they will act in their best interests in a particular circumstance, e.g. surgery. We will come back to consent later.

Truth-telling may be intrinsically good for the service user

Telling service users the truth may contribute generally to their health and well-being. For example, giving information prior to surgery has been shown to reduce anxiety and post-operative pain and improve recovery (see, for example, the seminal works of Boore, 1978; Hayward, 1975). Also, some people will simply find comfort in knowing that their symptoms can be attributed to a particular condition.

As one of the foundations of trust in the therapeutic relationship

If the service user's expectations of being told the truth are met then this will contribute to their trust in those responsible for their care (which we have already seen to be fundamental to the therapeutic relationship). Consequently, they may also be more willing to co-operate with and seek treatment when required.

Is it ever right to withhold the truth?

> deception is the real enemy of trust.
>
> (O'Neill, 2002d, p.3)

We generally believe that to deliberately deceive another, which includes withholding or distorting the truth or lying, is wrong. It is not just about getting the information wrong (which affects a person's ability to be autonomous) but is also about the motive and deliberate intention behind the deceit that is harmful to the person and their trust. If, in all honesty, you give the wrong directions to a stranger, they will find it annoying but not as much as if you had deliberately misled them for some personal pleasure or ends (O'Neill, 2002d, pp.3–4). Think about how you feel when someone has deliberately deceived you as a practical joke. A common joke when we trained as nurses was to be told to go 'for a long stand for a drip' (and you would be left standing in a particular place for a while before you realised that they didn't want an intravenous infusion stand at all). Alternatively, how would you feel if someone you secretly adored arranged to meet you for a date but never had any intention of turning up. In either case, you can imagine the humiliation, hurt, embarrassment, disbelief and anger that you might feel and it could well threaten your trust in the person that deceived you. As O'Neill (2002d, p.4) reminds us:

It is because their falsehood is deliberate, and because it implies a deliberate intention to undermine, damage or distort others' plans and their capacities to act, that it damages trust and future relationships.

(O'Neill, 2002d, p.4)

From this you can see the close connections with the value of respect for persons and their autonomy because the deception and misinformation frustrate a person's ability to be autonomous. Being untruthful, evading the truth, deception and lying can also have serious consequences, both in the direct harm to the individual and through damaging their trust in therapeutic relationships or those with relatives and carers. Thus, the different obligations related to truth-telling are:

• not to lie;
• not to deceive;
• to tell the truth.

To tell the truth appears, on the face of it, to be straightforward, although we could debate what the truth is in itself and certainly, in the current information age, the truth is becoming increasingly hard to know. It may be difficult to assess the 'truth' that should be told because of misleading or conflicting information. Take the example of the MMR vaccination: who should you believe? Who has authority among the proliferation of papers and contested claims in the evidence? Sometimes too much information can be as disabling as too little when attempting to make informed choices and decisions. However, it is essential that you keep up to date with the available evidence related to your practice and learn skills in literature reviewing and discriminating between the validity and reliability of sources, particularly the plethora of information on the internet, so that you can support service users who have difficulty in determining the authority and credibility of information. Of course, we may not always know the truth ourselves or be able to communicate the truth because of someone's incapacity to understand but this does not mean that you cannot still be truthful. To say, 'we don't know what is causing your symptoms' is being truthful (assuming this really is the case) even though it may not be what the person wants or needs to hear, and would be better than evading the fact that we don't know.

These truth-telling obligations may also become blurred in practice, particularly in cases where the truth seems potentially hurtful or when caring for people who lack mental capacity and the ability to distinguish between truths and falsehoods.

Imaginative exercise

Truth-telling and the person with dementia

Read the following two examples taken from Schermer (2007, pp.14--15).

Imagine a demented woman banging on the locked door of the ward, begging everyone in the neighbourhood to open the door so that she can go and collect the children from school. Telling her that her children are long grown up and are not waiting for her only worsens her agitation and confusion. So one of the nursing aides takes her arm and says, 'come on Mrs G, the children will not be out for another hour, let's go have a cup of tea first'. (p.14)

Another example is that of a widower who keeps asking about his wife, and who is inconsolable every time he is told that she has passed away. Why hurt such a patient by confronting him with the painful truth time and again? Why not just distract attention by a small lie and tell the widower his wife is out shopping? (pp.14--15)

1. What are your feelings about the suggested lying and deception in each of these hypothetical cases?

2. Is lying justified? Explain your answers.

We cannot ignore the fact that to act in this way is an act of lying, which is generally wrong, although the motive behind the lies and deception in each of these cases is (hopefully) one of avoiding harm and concern for the person's welfare (rather than one of self-interest, i.e. just making the job easier). There may also be some concomitant concerns for the welfare of others if the individual's behaviour is disturbing other patients, although careful consideration must be given as to whether this justifies lying to one individual for the benefit of others. Schermer (2007) argues that dementia slowly diminishes the capacities a person needs to distinguish between truths and falsehoods and, with this, the ability to be lied to also disappears. However, outright lies to people with dementia should be avoided because they compromise the practitioner as well as threaten to undermine trust in care services. If we believe lying is fundamentally wrong (imagine what we would do if we thought everyone might lie), the moral reasons to reject lying should apply equally for people with dementia. This may, however, depend on the capacities of the patient such that lying may sometimes be justified on the count of caring for their well-being. Remember, to say something is 'just a little white lie' makes no difference; it is still a euphemism for lying (but trying to convey perhaps that the motive is not bad). As with many moral dilemmas, there are no easy, straightforward answers but 'in general, methods that enhance the well-being of the patient without deception or lies should be favoured above options that use deceit, and methods of getting the truth across without hurting the patient should be favoured above blunt honesty' (Schermer, 2007, p.13).

Should you protect service users from 'bad news'?

Any justification for deception or evading the truth becomes even harder to establish in cases where the service user is fully competent and autonomous. Protecting the patient or service user from 'bad news' such as, for example, a diagnosis of chronic or terminal illness, even from a well-intentioned concern for their welfare, would be paternalistic, i.e. acting in what you assumed to be their best interests even when they were capable of autonomous decision-making. We have discussed some of the problems associated with paternalism in Chapter 3. Another argument sometimes mounted against truth-telling is that some patients and service users do not want to know the whole truth about their condition or prognosis because they would find it too burdensome. In cases where they are obviously autonomous and state their preference not to be told, it seems only right to allow them this choice and we should not force unwanted information on them (although lack of information to inform understanding and decisions may cause problems for informed consent). However, there is often a false assumption that patients do not or would not wish to be told the truth, even if it is unpleasant. Others may not ask but simply expect to be told more about their condition. One of the other difficulties is that one person's right to know or be told the truth may conflict with another person's right to confidentiality. For example, in cases of predictive genetic testing for Huntington's disease, someone may choose to be tested because their grandparent has the disease but their own parent has chosen not to be tested. However, if the test proves the grandchild has the faulty gene, then this automatically means that their parent has it as well. Trying then to keep this result secret is likely to be difficult or even impossible for the person who has been tested.

Reading activity

1. Locate and read the following journal article:

Anthony Tuckett's (2004) 'Truth-telling in clinical practice and the arguments for and against: a review of the literature.' *Nursing Ethics*, 11 (5): pp.500–13

> While reading, make notes that identify the arguments for and against truth-telling presented by Tuckett's review of the literature.
>
> 2. Do you agree with each of the arguments?
>
> 3. Can you think of additional arguments? If so, add these to your for-and-against list.

Lies and deceptions may be used with the best intentions. However, it is important to first seek other ways of conveying the truth, rather than resorting to using lies and deceit as the first line of action, to avoid hurting the service user. To do this will require good interpersonal and communication skills and insight into the individual's understanding, capacity and circumstances and the range of alternatives available in any given situation. The risk associated with getting into the habit of being economical with the truth, deceiving or lying is that you will too easily resort to these practices when they are not justified.

Trust, truth-telling and informed consent

Completing the next activity should help you to consolidate your thoughts on the rights and wrongs of truth telling and deception, and to start to think about the importance of consent as an expression of service user's trust.

Case study

Mary is a 79-year-old resident in the care home where you work as a care assistant. She has asthma that is generally well controlled. Recently, she developed a chest infection and has been prescribed two courses of antibiotics. However, although she recognises that the antibiotics are for her benefit, they are making her feel particularly unwell, with constant nausea and diarrhoea. When you and the care home manager take her the next dose of antibiotic, she refuses to take it, saying 'I can't take any more of these horrible things. Surely I have had enough of them by now. My family are visiting tomorrow, bringing my new grandson, and I don't want to feel lousy'. You both try to encourage her to take the tablets, but she continues to refuse them.

The manager is concerned. She knows the importance of giving the antibiotics at the prescribed intervals and that Mary should finish the course of medication, particularly as her asthma has been less well controlled since having the chest infection. She asks you to conceal the medication in Mary's food; she feels that it is more important that she has the antibiotics as she is fearful that she will develop pneumonia.

1. What should you do? Think about the arguments for and against truth-telling that you have already noted in the previous exercise. Is deception through the covert administration of medication justified in this case? Explain your answers.

Giving medication to a patient or service user normally requires their consent.

2. Why should you obtain consent?

3. What are the moral justifications for informed consent?

4. Can Mary refuse the medication as part of the consent process?

5. Are there any instances where consent would not be required?

The covert administration of medication is a controversial issue, particularly in cases where individuals are autonomous and have the capacity to make their own choices about what is right for them. There is no reason, from the information given here, to question Mary's capacity using the criteria in the Mental Capacity Act 2005. She has made a decision and has given a perfectly reasonable justification for it, based on her knowledge and experience of the effects of the medication. On this basis, she has the right to refuse the medication, even though her refusal may not concur with what others believe is in her overall best interests. You must respect her refusal just as much as you would her consent. If you disguise the medication in her food or drink, she is being led to believe that she is not receiving medication, when in fact she is. This is an obvious case of deception, although the manager's motive in doing so is generally well-intentioned, depending on how you view the balance of harms associated with her chest infection versus the discomfort and distress caused by the side-effects of the antibiotics. On balance, the better course of action would be to ask her GP if the antibiotics could be changed to avoid the side-effects. As a care assistant you have also been put in a difficult position because if you do as you have been asked, you would be held responsible for covertly administering the medication (although the manager would be accountable for her instruction to you). If Mary realises what you have both done, this could cause her distress and could easily destroy any relationship of trust you have with her and subsequently impact on her health and welfare. If she tells other residents, they too may become suspicious, lose faith and trust in your actions and feel a sense of abandonment by those who should be caring for them.

The following Nursing and Midwifery Council guideline, although obviously aimed at registered practitioners, provides insight into the main issues surrounding covert administration of medication and consent (including people who lack capacity and children):

The NMC position statement on the covert administration of medicines – disguising medicine in food and drink (NMC, 2006, at **www.nmc-uk.org/ aFrameDisplay.aspx?DocumentID=3397** (accessed 23 November 2007) or in their A–Z advice at **www.nmc-uk.org/aSection.aspx?SectionID=11 #sectionD** (accessed 23 November 2007). You would be advised to check their A-Z Advice listing at **www.nmc-uk.org** for any updated versions of this document.

INFORMED CONSENT

There is much written about the duty of informed consent, particularly in relation to the legal requirements for consent and the processes by which explicit consent should be obtained by medical practitioners or other professionals authorised to gain consent for specific, discrete medical examinations, procedures, surgery and investigations. Much of this kind of practice would be beyond the roles and responsibilities of a practitioner who is not a member of a registered or regulated profession. However, consent is a necessary part of any care relationship and all contact, including care procedures and interventions with service users, should be subject to a framework of informed choice and consent. As we are particularly concerned in this book with understanding values for practice, we will finish here on the moral justifications for consent, although these inevitably underpin much of what is understood from a legal or professional perspective.

What is the value associated with informed consent?

Consent can be simply defined as giving someone permission or authority to do something that they would not otherwise have the right to do without the individual's permission. The right of service users to give or to refuse consent is a prime way of expressing and exercising their autonomy, and giving their consent to care, interventions and treatment is the ultimate expression of their trust in another.

Informed consent is one hallmark of trust between strangers. For example, when I understand a pension plan, a mortgage, or complex medical procedures, and am free to choose or refuse, I express my trust by giving informed consent. We give informed consent in face-to-face transactions too, though we barely notice it.

We buy apples in the market, we exchange addresses with acquaintances, we sit down for a haircut. It sounds pompous to speak of these daily transactions as based on informed consent: yet in each we assume that the other party is neither deceiving nor coercing. We withdraw our trust very fast if we are sold rotten apples, or deliberately given a false address, or forcibly subjected to a Mohican haircut.

(O'Neill, 2002d, p.1)

Informed consent is not the basis of trust but occurs as a result of having trust in another, as an expression of our trust; i.e. a person must already trust you in order to give their consent. They may rely on you to provide accurate and reliable information, and on 'experts' to help them to assess the quality and effectiveness of interventions, but they have to already trust these people not to deceive them or have bad intentions. The ways in which they have arrived at this trust relate to the discussions at the beginning of this chapter and also as a result of their various experiences of the care relationship, such as whether or not their confidences have been respected. Informed consent is important because:

- of the value attributed to respect for persons and respect for their autonomy;
- having to obtain consent offers protection of the service user from harm (or at least unwarranted or uninvited harms);
- of a principle of concern for their welfare and best interests;
- it fosters trust and confidence;
- it promotes service user responsibility for their health and well-being;
- of the protection it affords the practitioner;
- it is required by law.

Consent and the value of respect for persons and respect for their autonomy

You have already seen in Chapter 2 that respect for persons is a fundamental value in health and social care and that people should be supported and enabled to be self-determining. Being autonomous also means there is an expectation that people will take control of, and be responsible for, their own lives. Consent is therefore essential to any duty of respect for autonomy and self-determination. Consent involves the service user making (and taking responsibility for) their own choices regarding what does, or does not, happen to them. To touch a person without their consent is a form of trespass on their person which is a harm. All of the factors that are required in order to be autonomous (and those that can prevent people from being autonomous) that have already been discussed, in this chapter and in Chapter 3, apply to the consent process.

Therefore, the general requirements for informed consent come from the following expectations and necessary conditions for autonomy.

- The person has the capacity or competence to understand, express their preferences, make choices and decisions.
- The person has freedom from overwhelming influences or interferences (such as manipulation and coercion). This is often referred to as voluntariness or making voluntary choices and decisions (this includes the freedom to say 'no' or refuse or withhold consent).
- Disclosure of adequate and accurate information and having an understanding of this information as a basis for their decision-making (which includes time to consider and deliberate their options).
- Consent also requires that a decision is made.

Informed consent can therefore be defined as:

> a voluntary, uncoerced decision, made by a sufficiently competent or autonomous person on the basis of adequate information and deliberation, to accept rather than reject some proposed course of action that will affect him or her.
>
> (Gillon, 1986, p.113)

Whenever possible, it is important to treat obtaining consent as a process, not a one-off event. Service users often need time to think through the options and consequences of their decisions before arriving at their final decision. They are also free to change their minds and withdraw consent at any time. If there is any doubt, you should always check that they still consent to you caring for or treating them.

Consent and concern for their welfare and best interests

If, in seeking consent, we are concerned with enabling the service user to be self-determining, we should also assume that the competent person will be the best judge of what is in their best interests. Although practitioners may have knowledge and expertise that can be used to help inform the service user of the best treatment or intervention, they may not be the best judge of other factors that matter equally (or more importantly) to the service user such as, for example, those factors arising from their particular cultural or religious background. You must be careful not to judge the service user's decisions according to what you would want for yourself or to manipulate their decision in order to ensure that it concurs with what you determine to be in their best interest. However, you may help them understand that certain courses of action may result in better outcomes (if this is truly the case), although the requirement to provide adequate information means that this should also be balanced (i.e. you identify both the harms and benefits).

> The provision of sufficient accurate information is an essential part of seeking consent. Acquiescence when a patient does not know what the intervention entails, or is unaware that he or she can refuse, is not 'consent'. Consent is a process, not a one-off event, and it is important that there is continuing discussion to reflect the evolving nature of treatment.
>
> (BMA, 2007)

Service users who are fully informed about, and involved in, the decisions about their care may also be more likely to trust the practitioner and co-operate and participate in their care, hence contributing to their overall well-being. (See Figure 4.5 for guidance on helping someone make a decision for themselves.)

To help someone make a decision for themselves, check the following points.

Providing relevant information:

- Does the person have all the relevant information they need in order to make a particular decision?
- If they have a choice, have they been given information on all the alternatives?

Communicating in an appropriate way:

- Could information be explained or presented in a way that is easier for the person to understand (for example, by using simple language or visual aids)?
- Have different methods of communication been explored if required, including non-verbal communication?
- Could anyone else help with communication (for example, a family member, support worker, interpreter, speech and language therapist or advocate)?

Making the person feel at ease:

- Are there particular times of day when the person's understanding is better?
- Are there particular locations where they may feel more at ease?
- Could the decision be put off to see whether the person can make the decision at a later time when circumstances are right for them?

Supporting the person:

- Can anyone else help or support the person to make choices or express a view?

Figure 4.5 Helping someone to make a decision for themselves (from the *Mental Capacity Act 2005 Code of Practice* (DCA, 2007, p.29)

Consent – what is required by law?

The requirement in law for obtaining consent is based principally on the right of competent individuals to self-determination. There is no English statute setting out the general principles of consent (other than that related to the Mental Capacity Act (2005)). The requirement for consent is based instead in the common law (case law), which has established the offence of battery if a person is touched without their valid consent. Consent may be either explicit or implied.

- **Explicit consent** – (sometimes called *express consent*) is usually given orally or in writing and conveys a clear indication of the individual's preference or choice (which may be in relation to a specific intervention or aspect of care). The choice or decision should be made freely or voluntarily in light of knowledge of the available options and the consequences.
- **Implied consent** – is where a service user or patient's agreement to a course of action has been demonstrated by their behaviour; for example, when they offer their arm freely for blood pressure monitoring. However, care must be taken not to make assumptions of implied consent and it should still meet the necessary conditions, such that you are confident that the individual genuinely knows and understands what is being proposed on the basis of adequate information.

Both forms of consent are equally relevant in the law, although it is easier to validate explicit consent, particularly if written. Failure to gain proper consent for an intervention that later causes the service user harm may be used in claims of negligence. Poor consent processes may also result in complaints, either through employers or professional bodies (or both). Written explicit consent is usually supported by appropriate documentation provided by organisations, such as that provided by the Department of Health. However, much of the consent you will obtain for everyday care interventions will be either verbal or implied. Thus, it is particularly important that you maintain accurate records of care and document where explicit verbal consent has been given and the process used to establish consent prior to care interventions.

For a detailed legal explanation and exploration of issues related to consent see, for example, Dimond (2004, Chapter 7), Jackson (2006, Chapters 4 and 5) or Hendrick (2004, Chapter 6). Note, however, that, as with any aspect of law, you should seek out the most up-to-date edition of any textbook to ensure it reflects current legal and professional practice. The Mental Capacity Act 2005 (DCA, 2005) and its Code of Practice (DCA, 2007) are also essential sources when determining a person's capacity to give or withhold their consent. Other good sources of professional guidance (and whose principles are transferable to care practice) include the British Medical Association Consent Tool Kit (2007), professional codes of conduct or practice (for example, NMC, 2004; GSCC, 2002) and the Department of Health Good Practice in Consent initiative, details of which can be accessed from their website at **www.dh.gov.uk/en/ Policyandguidance/Healthandsocialcaretopics/Consent/index.htm** (accessed 22 November 2007). This includes guidance on meeting the specific needs of a range of service users in the consent process, including children and young people, older people and people with learning disabilities.

CONCLUSION

Learning to be trustworthy may not be as straightforward as it sounds. It is more than being reliable and skilled to perform tasks or a role to some defined standard. It also requires you to develop a trustworthy disposition, with sensitivity to the values of the service user and insight into the value they attribute to what they entrust to you, be it their personal and intimate information, their well-being, support or whatever else. It is essential that you take responsibility for the effect you have on their perception of trust both in you and, as a consequence, in other practitioners. It is also vital that you do not exploit the vulnerability and good will of the service user when they place their trust in you. Practising in ways that preserve and protect service users' privacy through your duty of confidentiality, being honest and not deceitful in your interpersonal interactions and respecting their autonomous choices through the consent process in care decisions, are all ways in which you can foster trustworthiness and justify the trust service users place in you.

SUMMARY OF KEY POINTS

- Building successful care relationships with service users and patients depends on trust.
- Trust and trustworthiness can be understood in a number of ways, including as an attitude towards other people or as a characteristic of individuals that can be described in moral terms and as a virtue.
- Maintaining confidentiality is one of the fundamental principles for trust in care practice. There are strong moral justifications, including respect for individual autonomy, promoting patient welfare and maintaining trust in the care relationship.
- Breaching confidentiality can be morally justified, or even required in some circumstances, i.e. in the best interests of the service user, in the public interest or when required by law. However, any breach should be exceptional and, if a decision is made to breach patient confidentiality, the service user must be informed.

- Trust is generally promoted by honesty and truth-telling or undermined by deception; exceptions are rarely justified.
- One of the real expressions of a patient's or service user's trust is when they give informed consent for you to perform a procedure or do something on their behalf.

FURTHER READING

Butterworth, C. (2005) 'Ongoing consent to care for older people in care homes', *Nursing Standard,* 19(20): 40–5

De Raeve, L. (2002) 'Trust and trustworthiness in nurse-patient relationships', *Nursing Philosophy*, 3: 152–62

Department of Constitutional Affairs/Ministry of Justice (2007) *Mental Capacity Act 2005. Code of Practice*. London: The Stationery Office

Department for Educational and Skills (2005) *Common Core of Skills and Knowledge for the Children's Workforce*. Nottingham: DfES Publications

Department of Health (2003) *NHS Code of Practice for Confidentiality*. London: The Stationery Office

O'Neill, O. (2002) *A Question of Trust. The BBC Reith Lectures 2002* Cambridge: Cambridge University Press, or available as transcripts at **www.bbc.co.uk/radio4/reith2002/lectures.shtml** (accessed 26 October 2007)

Partners in Care (2004) *Carers and confidentiality in mental health. Issues involved in information-sharing*. London: Royal College of Psychiatrists, at **www.rcpsych.ac.uk/campaigns/partnersincare.aspx** (accessed 29 October 2007)

Sellman, D. (2006) 'The importance of being trustworthy', *Nursing Ethics*, 13 (2): 105–15

Chapter 5

Protection from Harm and Promoting Independence

Key themes

In this chapter you will:

- consider the duty of care in protecting clients;

- reflect on the concept of risk;

- apply the principles of risk assessment and risk management to the care context;

- consider the value of independence;

- apply the notion of planned risk-taking to the care context.

INTRODUCTION

Protection from harm and the promotion of independence are central values for care work. The GSCC *Code of Practice for Care Workers* (GSCC, 2002) requires care workers to 'protect the independence of service users while protecting them as far as possible from danger or harm'. These core values arise out of the 'duty of care' that is owed to the recipient of care by anyone who is contracted to protect their interests and to provide a care service. Service users should be protected from harm and should not be worse off as a result of care than they were before they received it. Protection from harm is clearly implicit within the 'duty of care'. What is less clear is the duty to promote independence. However, overprotection and failure to promote improvement and independence are harmful. Therefore, independence is an important component of the duty of care. Of course, in order to promote independence, it is necessary to take risks and when you take risks there is always the possibility that you will sustain harm. Thus, the care worker must constantly balance the competing demands of care that is neither overprotective nor too risky, and which does promote independence.

The promotion of best interests

Protection from harm has been a long-standing responsibility of practitioners who provide care. In the past the articulation of this principle of protection from harm was frequently interpreted as 'the promotion of best interests'. That is, that the practitioner would determine best interests on behalf of the patient, usually based upon what would be best for their physical recovery or rehabilitation. This focus arose out of the primacy of the 'medical model of care' that suggested that practitioners, doctors in particular, knew what was in the best interests of those in their care, and that they were best placed to action those best interests. Inevitably this led to a paternalistic or parental approach to care practice, in which the practitioner had licence to tell the client what to do, and to expect that the client would comply with those directions. Increasingly, this approach to care practice has come to be seen as problematic. The reasons for this are that this approach has a tendency to identify people by their illness or disability and care is consequently focused on that aspect of the person, rather than care that is designed to meet the many and varied needs and preferences of individuals, some of which may have nothing to do with the service user's physical health. If care is focused on illness rather than on individuals, it is difficult to accommodate individual differences and preferences.

While the 'best interests' approach to care has fallen out of favour in recent times, it is important to note that it is not always an inappropriate approach to select, as long as it is selected with caution and an appropriate rationale. It is easy to accept that there are times when an individual is too weak, or too compromised, to make decisions for themselves about their care and they may ask you to act in their best interests. There are also times when, where safety is concerned, best interests, in the form of paternalism, is the fundamental reason for undertaking an action that protects someone from danger. What is important is that the best-interests approach, which favours a paternalistic stance, should be used only with appropriate justification. Practitioners should be constantly alert to the service user's rights to take back control of the decision-making in care at any point or as soon as they are able to do so.

Increasingly our understanding of care is being challenged by significant philosophical and social changes that require practitioners to engage with service users as different, unique individuals for whom one rule of care cannot be applied. This social change is clearly reflected in government policy, which promotes the idea of independence and choice in care such as *Choosing health: making healthy choices easier* (DoH, 2004a) and *Independence, well-being and choice* (DoH, 2005b). In addition, we are living in an increasingly risk-averse society in which the fulfilment of rights, while also being protected from risks, has become a significant expectation.

This chapter will explore the concepts of protection from harm and the promotion of independence within the context of an increasingly risk-aware and risk-averse society. In addition, the chapter will seek to provide practical examples of how care workers can both protect from harm and promote independence.

WHAT IS RISK AND DO WE NEED TO BE PROTECTED FROM IT?

Risks are part of our everyday experience; it is hard to imagine any activity that does not involve an element of risk. We learn from a very early age about risk assessment and risk taking. Initially this might be simplistic and might not be done at a conscious level. For example, children constantly test boundaries with their parents and risk censure in order to see what they can get away with. In this way they learn how to make judgements about activities. Similarly, as adolescents and adults, we continue to learn from our experiences and from acquiring knowledge. We develop a bank of information that we can draw upon to help us make decisions when we face the same, similar or new situations in the future. When we are exposed to opportunities and experiences that we have never encountered before, we make some assessment of the activity and decide whether or not this is a risk that we want to take. Without engaging in risk taking it is impossible to become independent. Therefore, the notions of risk and independence are inextricably linked.

Defining risk

Although risk-taking behaviours are, and always have been, part of our everyday lives, and although risk is essential for growth and development, risk and risk management have become a preoccupation and, some would say, the dominating feature of life in the twenty-first century (Denney, 2005) and yet there is no real consensus on the definition of risk.

The word 'risk' has been traced back to its early Arabic origin, *risq*, a term used to denote outcomes that can be either positive or negative (Alaszewski *et al.*, 1998). However, by the time 'risk' became part of the English language in the fifteenth century it had taken on a purely negative connotation and was primarily linked to the idea of hazards:

the possibility of an objective danger an act of God, or a *force majeure*.

(Lupton, 1999, p.5)

The fact that these hazards were seen to be beyond human control, i.e. acts of God or fate, meant that although they needed to be noted, primarily so that insurance in losses to shipping cargoes could be determined, no other preventative action was needed. Even though risk was understood as a negative thing, it was tolerated as a natural part of life. In recent years, risk has come to be seen as something that should be predicted, prevented, avoided or managed.

Why are we so risk-conscious?

There are a number of theories about why our attitude to risk has changed so radically in recent years, for example:

- we are exposed to more risks now than in the past, and that these risks are of a more devastating nature (Beck, 1992);
- the knowledge revolution now means that we have the knowledge to understand and prevent risks in a way not possible in previous times;
- the increasingly secular society means that we can no longer blame God for what happens to us, but must be reliant on our own resources;
- the individualisation of Western societies means that we must be responsible for our own actions and behaviours.

Whatever the reason, we are constantly bombarded by warnings of the need to be aware of risks and to act responsibly. The daily reminders of risks regarding global warming; terrorism; the dangers of speeding; of sunbathing; of eating too much, getting fat and of taking too little exercise; of the vulnerability of children, etc., are endless and all give us the impression that life has become dangerous, that risks are bad and that we must take precautions and avoid risks; that wherever possible we should be adopting the 'better safe than sorry' principle (Furedi, 1997).

While much of this is good advice and can to some extent explain why we enjoy healthier, longer lives than ever before, it would be a mistake to believe that risk can, or should, be eliminated. What has been lost in the modern understanding of risk is the idea of positive outcomes.

Reflection

Remember a time when you took a risk in order to do something that you really wanted to do. Perhaps it was riding on a particularly high roller coaster, or driving on your own for the first time, or skiing down a steep mountain or risking doing a performance in front of an audience or when you attempted something you never thought you could do. Whatever the activity you have in mind, remember the thrill and excitement of undertaking that activity, remember the sense of achievement and self-belief when that activity went well.

Risk taking can be thrilling and taking risks frequently does have a positive outcome. Without risk life would be boring, humans would cease to grow and to develop. If you apply this idea to the context of health many of the positive outcomes in terms of treatments and advances in medicine have only occurred because someone took a risk.

Risk in health and social care

Why is all this relevant to the care worker? In protecting those in our care from harm, it is all too easy to focus on the negative side of risk. This inevitably causes us to practise in a defensive manner, which causes us to err on the side of caution. For example, we may seek to restrict the free movement of someone who has been known to fall but, while this may keep them safe, it fails to acknowledge their right to independence and to take risks; overprotection means that their mobility may deteriorate still further and their confidence and sense of self-esteem may be seriously affected. In this case the care worker can consider a number of questions relating to the key question: 'In what ways can I assist this person to more safely maintain their independent mobility?' After all, it might be necessary to acknowledge that absolute safety is unrealistic and that suitable preventative activities to reduce risk are the only really appropriate methods of addressing the issue. Therefore, the questions to ask might be:

- Does the individual have appropriately supportive shoes?
- Are there any walking aids that would offer support but enable the person to retain their independence?
- Is the environment safe?
- Are there any unnecessary obstacles that hinder the individual's mobility?
- Could the individual be offered an assessment with a physiotherapist to learn some strategies for greater stability?

These are just some of the strategies that can be explored. It may be easier to protect the individual, but the real care emerges from looking at the problem and trying to find solutions not to eliminate the risk, but to manage the risk more effectively.

At times risk assessment is undertaken at an organisational level and results in the development of a policy in relation to a specific issue.

> **Example**
>
> An organisation, providing full-time care for adolescents, may have a policy requiring all 16-year-olds and younger to be in by 21.00 hours.
>
> How should the care worker respond to a request from a responsible 16-year-old to stay out later than the 21.00 hours deadline?

The care worker may be convinced of the safety of the request in this case, but is constrained by the policy because it has been assessed that imposing a curfew is an appropriate risk-management strategy. In this instance the care worker may need to comply with the policy, but undertake to challenge that policy through discussion with managers and the adolescents themselves. Risk assessments cannot be made in isolation from the context in which we operate, and at times there are things that we cannot challenge. What is important is not to follow policies blindly but to engage actively with them, in order to see if they are still 'fit for purpose'.

The fear of blame

The risk focus in our society today is largely motivated by fear of blame. Part of our risk assessment will entail an analysis such as the following: 'if I let this activity go ahead, what will happen if I have made a poor judgement and something goes wrong?' These worries may be partly on behalf of the person in our care, but equally may be worries about ourselves. 'If I make the wrong decision, will I be blamed? What will happen to me?' The increasing threat of being sued has resulted in an ever-increasing number of policies that effectively reduce the opportunities for individual practitioners to take independent decisions. Some of this is beyond our control and is a reflection of the society we live in. However, it is a useful exercise when we seek to protect, particularly in respect of restricting others' activities and freedom, to think about these questions:

- Who am I protecting and why?
- Is the level of restriction appropriate?
- Are there any other ways to manage the issue?

The growth of policy is part of the wider governance agenda that seeks to improve standards and protect those in our care through the better control and standardisation of the behaviours of practitioners.

Governance is the response of the health and care sector to a series of public scandals in the health and social care arenas. Governance is also driven by an increasingly knowledgeable, but cynical, public whose expectations are significantly higher than they were 20 years ago, and who will seek compensation for errors of judgement. Governance is therefore an attempt to reassure the public of the safety and efficacy of the services that are provided. Risk assessment and risk management are a central element of that process. A central theme of governance is to develop a culture in which organisations and individuals are able to look at risk proactively. This is to ensure that good policies and procedures are in place to protect individuals and prevent accidents from happening, to analyse accidents to learn from mistakes and improve policies and procedures, and to create a culture of openness that encourages individuals to admit their mistakes and errors. This can only be achieved if an organisation is able to convey the message that the investigation of mistakes is not to apportion blame but rather to learn from mistakes.

RISK ASSESSMENT

Risk assessment is now a daily activity within the care sector and is a key feature of protecting our clients from harm. Risk assessment requires a practitioner to think through the consequences of their decision-making and their actions and make judgements on the basis of this activity. When engaging in risk assessment, practitioners are encouraged to assess the nature of the risk posed, as different types of risks need to be treated in different ways.

Predictable and preventable risks

Risks that are predictable, likely to be frequent and/or avoidable are issues that require us to put preventative strategies in place. These strategies may be seen as 'good house-keeping'. These risks should be anticipated and changes in practice should be implemented to prevent or reduce their incidence. An example of dealing with this type of risk are measures to try to protect service users from acquired infections. Procedures for hand-washing and the widespread introduction of alcohol hand-rubs are measures that have been introduced to reduce a known and frequent risk.

Risk assessment leading to 'policy implementation' is also used as a means to protect individuals from infrequent but potentially significant harm such as, for example, fire safety procedures. All organisations have well-established policies and procedures that would come into play in the unfortunate event of a fire. Staff are trained in the implementation of the policy on a regular basis, even though many will never have to put it into practice. However, the training and knowing what to do if a fire happened could save lives so it is therefore an investment worth making.

Assessing individual risk

Risk assessment can also be applied to individual situations – assessing individual risk. This may be a one-off or a regular activity that relates to a specific person or group of service users. Assessing individual risks should be part of the day-to-day planning and care of people. However, the mind-set that the practitioner adopts in relation to risk assessment will determine what decisions will come out of the assessment. If the practitioner sees danger in situations that are not completely within their control, then they are likely to risk-assess in a defensive and restrictive manner, and may decide not to engage in an activity at all. This is certainly what has happened in relation to the provision of school trips: because of a few widely publicised problems that have occurred, teachers are increasingly reluctant to arrange trips, believing that abstaining from them is the most appropriate preventative strategy.

However, if the practitioner approaches risk assessment from a positive perspective, seeing risk as an essential part of life that must be engaged with and managed, then the risk assessment and the strategies that ensue from that will mean that the activity is less likely to be prevented and may be conducted in a safer manner than if no risk assessment had been made.

Reflection

1. Plan a trip/visit out with someone in your care. What risks do you think you are likely to expose the client to? Are there risks to you? Are there risks to others?

2. Can any of the risks be reduced?

Doing a risk assessment is very likely to throw up all manner of potential risks and might discourage the care worker from engaging in the activity. However, it is very important to be able to distinguish between real risks and possible but unlikely risks (virtual risks). Remember what it feels like to take risks and to do the things that you really want to do. If you enjoy the sensation of risk taking then so too will the person in your care. Taking reasonable and well thought-through risks with service users is likely to give you, and them, a positive sense of achievement, but will also provide them with an opportunity to experience those things that bring quality to life. Living a life that is completely predictable and one hundred per cent protected is a very depressing thought. If viewed as a positive opportunity for safe practice, risk-taking may enhance the care of individuals and consequently enhance their life.

Writing activity

From your own experience, list examples of:

- risks that are managed through 'good house-keeping';
- policies that exist to combat infrequent, but significant, potential risk;
- risk assessment of individual client issues.

The fact that a risk is likely or that a risk could have significant impact does not necessarily mean that we should not engage in the risk. However it does of course mean that additional care needs to be taken and the activity needs to be planned in order that the risk is minimised to an acceptable level and individuals and organisations are reasonably protected.

PREDICTING RISK

It should be noted that many risks are very difficult to predict accurately (Gale *et al.*, 2003; Titterton, 2005). It is commonly assumed that risk can be predicted through the application of objective assessment, reasoning about evidence and the prediction of likelihood and probability. However, risk assessment is not simply a matter of calculating the likelihood of an action happening and assessing the likelihood and magnitude of the potential harm that could result from taking that risk.

Discussion activity

1. Think about the risks of the following in your own life and try to predict the probability of them actually happening. For example, winning the Lottery is well known to be a chance of somewhere in the region of 1:14 million.

- Being burgled.
- Getting Alzheimer's disease.
- Falling and breaking your leg.
- Being involved in an aeroplane crash.

2. Ask five other people the same questions. Discuss the similarities and differences in your answers. Can you identify any reasons for differences?

Some risks have been the subject of significant research and we can predict fairly accurately the incidence or possibility of an occurrence happening. For example, our knowledge of epidemiology will fairly accurately be able to identify the statistical risk of contracting a disease, whereas there is insufficient evidence to predict the likelihood of me falling and breaking my leg. However, the incidence of a disease in the population does not help me to understand what that risk really means to me. My understanding of the risk will depend on how well I understand numbers and ratios, statistics and probability. Even if I do understand the figures, my interpretation of them will depend on a variety of factors and will determine whether I see the risk as a deterrent or an encouragement. For example, I might be tempted to play the Lottery, because a 1:14 million chance is better than a 1:0 chance if I do not play. On the other hand, if the risk of 1:14 million applied to the risk of me contracting a disease, I would interpret that as being negligible and would not think that I needed to bother about it. However, someone else might see that as a real risk and take precautionary action. These differences in understanding and interpreting risks are known as risk perception.

Risk perception

The increasing concentration on risk in society has caused social scientists to explore the way in which individuals assess risk and what influences differences in people's perceptions of risk.

> Risk perception involves people's beliefs, attitudes, judgements, experiences, and feelings, as well as the wider social or cultural values and dispositions that people adopt, towards hazards and their benefits.
>
> (Pidgeon *et al.*, 1992, p.89)

A number of factors affect our risk assessment and subsequent behaviour.

- Our personality type – some people are naturally more cautious than others.
- Joffe (2003) asserts that individuals have an unrealistically optimistic belief that their future holds few adverse events.
- Women are generally less keen to take risks than men (Karakowsky and Elangovan, 2001).
- If an individual has positive feelings about a particular thing, because of past experience, personal values or unrealistic beliefs, then their risk assessment will be significantly different from someone who has negative feelings about a particular issue.
- Primacy – if there has been a great deal of publicity about a particular topic, or this is associated with very striking, disturbing or unpleasant

effects, this will normally inflate your assessment of the frequency of the risk occurring (think, for example, about your own risk assessment of catching bird flu). People tend to overemphasise death from infrequent causes like bird flu or BSE and underestimate their risk of death from frequent causes such as cancer or heart disease (Pidgeon *et al.*, 1992).

- Fear of blame is likely to cause an individual to overemphasise the risk involved in an action.
- Some persons are perceived to be at more risk than others – for example, children or the older person. Others are perceived to be more of a risk than others – for example, those with mental health problems or those that take drugs (Kemshall and Pritchard, 1996).
- The views of others – our notion of risk is impacted on by dominant beliefs and values in our culture and by those in our social groups and networks who will influence how we understand and relate to risk. This is known as the social construction of risk.

Differences in risk perception and individual responses to risk mean that any objective measurement of risk is only partially useful. It means that I am unlikely to make an accurate assessment of your preparedness to take a risk if I do not spend time finding out how you feel about an issue or how you interpret risk factors. The same applies to clients in our care. All too often, care workers make assumptions about what is best for individuals in their care without ever really discussing with them whether this is so. Risk cannot and should not be eliminated. What is relevant is ascertaining which risks are appropriate to take and in what way.

ASSESSING RISK IN PRACTICE

There are lots of different tools and proformas for assessing risk in practice, but they should all ask the practitioner to engage with questions similar to the following ones.

- Is the risk a real risk?
- Why is the risk activity proposed?
- Is there a good justification for the risk activity?
- What advantages are there of engaging in this activity?
- What could go wrong and for whom?
- How could this happen?
- What could the effect be?
- How severe will this effect be?
- How likely is it that this will happen?

Involving the service user in risk assessment

All of these questions will help to build up a picture of the costs and benefits of a particular activity. Ironically, risk assessment is seen as the domain and responsibility of the care worker. There is scant evidence in risk assessment literature of the active involvement of, and taking account of the views of, the service users themselves. However, you should, wherever possible, ask service users:

- What is the individual's/family's view of the risk?
- How important to the individual is taking this risk?
- How willing is the individual to risk a negative outcome?

Risk assessment requires practitioners to make judgements about another's capabilities, about the potential gains for the individual concerned, the potential disadvantages or harms of the risk, the values placed on the outcomes and the consequences of not going ahead with the risk (Titterton, 2005), but this cannot be done in isolation from the service user. Having made an assessment, the outcome of the assessment should be discussed with the service user and other members of the team to determine whether the risk should be engaged in and/or whether a risk plan can be put in place to take reasonable precautions to limit any negative outcome.

Using risk-assessment tools

Writing activity

Using the structured risk-assessment tool in Figure 5.1 (on pages 133–5), recalculate the risk assessment for taking a client out on a visit that you did as an activity earlier in this chapter. Has your risk assessment changed?

Risk-assessment tools do not necessarily provide the right answer. They are there to provide you with prompts to help to ensure that important issues for consideration have not been forgotten. Their use provides evidence of the assessment process that you have undertaken and demonstrates that you took the risks seriously. It should be remembered that accidents, mishaps and risks cannot be prevented. What is relevant is that we approach activities responsibly and with risks in mind so that we may be able to minimise the risks to which individuals are exposed.

Risk-assessment tool for managed positive risk-taking

Location/service user(s) name(s) as appropriate:

Date:

Assessor:

---

1. Brief description of activity/issue and rationale for why the risk activity is proposed.

---

2. What are the benefits of engaging in this activity and for whom?

---

3. What is the significance of each of the benefits? Rate them on a 1–5 score with 5 = very important and 1= not at all important. (Discuss the results w th other relevant staff and the client/family.)

Benefit	Significance
	1 2 3 4 5
	1 2 3 4 5
	1 2 3 4 5
	1 2 3 4 5

4. Who benefits, how do they benefit and how likely is the benefit?

Who might benefit?	How might they benefit?	How likely is the benefit? (1 = not at all likely to 5 = very likely)
		1 2 3 4 5
		1 2 3 4 5
		1 2 3 4 5
		1 2 3 4 5
		1 2 3 4 5

Total benefits score =

5. What risks/hazards could result from the activity? (Consider risks to the service user, the practitioner and the organisation.)

6. What is the significance of each of the risks/hazards? Rank them, with 1 being not very significant and 5 being very significant.

Risk	Significance
	1 2 3 4 5
	1 2 3 4 5
	1 2 3 4 5
	1 2 3 4 5

7. Who might be harmed, how might they be harmed and how likely are they to be harmed?

Who might be harmed?	How might they be harmed?	How likely is the harm? 1 = highly unlikely 3 = can be reasonably foreseen 5 = highly likely
		1 2 3 4 5
		1 2 3 4 5
		1 2 3 4 5
		1 2 3 4 5
		1 2 3 4 5
		1 2 3 4 5

Total risk score =

8. Compare the risks and benefits overall. Does either of the scores suggest that benefits outweigh risks or vice versa?

9. What (if any) strategies could be put in place to make the activity safer?

10. If these strategies are put in place, does this change the risk assessment score?

11. What is the overall score, having taken account of the effects of strategies that can be implemented to minimise the risks?
Benefits =   Risks =

12. Decision on action to be taken and reason for decision:

Signed:

Practitioner_____ Service user _____
                                        (or approved representative)

Figure 5.1 Risk-assessment tool for managed positive risk-taking

RISK MANAGEMENT AND PROTECTION FROM HARM

Risk management implies a sense of control over risk. It suggests that if we undertake the assessment properly and put appropriate strategies in place then the risk will no longer be an issue. First, this approach to life fails to recognise the uncertainty of risk and the inability to accurately predict exactly what is likely to happen and in what circumstances. Secondly, it starts from the belief that all risks should be managed. Attempting to assess risk might be a very useful exercise in ensuring that people think carefully through the potential consequences of their actions. However, it is not as easy to accept that because a potential risk has been identified it necessarily should be managed. Inevitably, concentration on risk identifies real risks but it is also likely to identify potential virtual risks that warrant no further action. The danger of risk assessment is that it inevitably leads us to move into trying to devise a plan for all risks identified, not just those that should be selected for our attention.

Risk management also runs the risk of paternalism and being too parental in relation to those in our care. Paternalism can, while being well meaning, be an abuse of power over those in care. While it is clear that care workers do owe service users a duty of care, and this includes a duty to protect them from harm, it does not provide care workers with a licence to over-ride others' wishes, beliefs and rights in the name of protection. Most of the service users in care, although they may be vulnerable, are perfectly capable and, in law, entitled to make decisions about their own lives, including the risks that they wish to engage in. Care workers are expected to care, to support, to help, even to advise, but not to control. For those very vulnerable people who do not have the capacity to make risk choices, the same process of assessment should be worked through, with the care worker trying, where possible, to reflect the service user's known views and involving family and other care workers. However, it is acknowledged that a greater level of protection might be desirable for those that are unable to express a preference.

The language of risk management is not well suited to the personal care of individuals because it causes us to take an unnecessarily negative approach to risk by assuming that risk management is only about prevention. If this is the interpretation, then risk management is best suited to the development of policy and systems at organisational level. Risk management is particularly well suited to the airline industry, for example, where failure to engage in risk management would have devastating consequences, and where the risk management itself results in relatively little inconvenience for passengers when compared with the increased safety that it offers. Of course, at organisational level in health and social care, risk management also fulfils an important role in protecting the public and promoting safety. However, the same cannot be said of the individual care environment where attention to risk and restriction of rights in relation to a potential harm may have a significant, negative impact on the individual.

Managed risk taking

Titterton (2005) proposes a move away from risk management and towards a managed risk-taking approach in the individual care environment. This does not mean that risks should not be assessed and explored but, rather, that risks are approached from a more positive perspective. Given that it is impossible to eliminate risk, and given the positive outcomes of risk taking, how can we enable the service user to engage in this risk, while appropriately protecting them from unnecessary harm? Titterton proposes a step approach to risk taking.

- **Consult and communicate** – this involves an opportunity for all interested parties to discuss their point of view.
- **Prepare a risk plan** – which identifies who has been consulted, what has been decided, who is responsible, timescales and how risk will be monitored and outcomes measured. It also includes what records will be kept.
- **Sign up** – all interested parties should sign and agree a risk plan.
- **Share information** – all involved must be fully informed.
- **Monitor and review** – even the best-laid plans may need reviewing.
- **Support staff** – when appropriate processes are in place and reasonable care has been taken, it is important that staff are supported, even if a negative outcome ensues. The point is not to blame but to try to find out why something happened, so that it can be anticipated in the future (Titterton, 2005, pp.93–5).

CONCLUSION

Independence and the ability to live life according to one's own preferences, beliefs and choices are important values in maintaining a good quality of life. Protecting an individual's right to independence is no less important than protecting an individual from harm. Consequently, it is important to teach practitioners how to support service users to engage in risk safely. Equally, organisations need to learn how to support practitioners in appropriate risk taking with those in their care. Risk management and the promotion of independence should be proactive. All too often they are reactive: we wait until something has happened and then we approach all other risks from a negative viewpoint. Either that or, because practitioners are frightened to take risks on behalf of their clients, they practise in a cautious and defensive manner. If, however, we address risk proactively, planned and positive risk taking is a more likely outcome.

A welcome emphasis on user involvement and the implementation of Expert Patient initiatives demonstrate admirably that service users do not relish being 'told what to do in their best interests'. It is a salutary thought that the risks taken by service users are their risks not ours, and that to deny them choice in the decision-making process is probably foolhardy and is definitely arrogant. However, that does not mean that the practitioner has no responsibility for the actions or the outcome.

Protection from harm and the promotion of independence are not necessarily contradictory; unless they are interpreted as absolutes. If an individual must be protected from all possible harm, it is very unlikely that one would wish to allow any independence. Alternatively, promoting absolute independence in a care relationship is likely to lead to charges of negligence. As with many of the decisions in care, each situation must be assessed on its own individual merits and as much information, from a number of relevant sources, must be taken into account in the decision-making process. However, what is important to remember is how much each of us values our opportunities to be independent and to take risks, as well as our need, at times, to be protected. No less should be afforded to those in our care.

Writing activity

In partnership with a client (or friend, if you are not working in a care environment) undertake a risk assessment for a particular activity and try to develop a risk plan that enables appropriate risk-taking.

SUMMARY OF KEY POINTS

This chapter has identified that care is no longer solely focused on what is in the best interests of the service user from a health perspective. Instead, care must take account of a number of different factors including:

- the need to treat people differently and to respect their individual differences and preferences;
- the promotion of independence;
- the need to anticipate and protect people from harm while not compromising independence unduly;
- a focus on risk prevention that leads to cautious and restrictive care.

This chapter suggests that risks are part of our everyday life and are necessary for our growth and development at all stages of our life. Consequently, it is suggested that managed risk-taking is part of the care decision-making process. A model has been provided to help practitioners engage with appropriate risk taking in the care setting.

FURTHER READING

Department of Health (2005) *Independence, wellbeing and choice: our vision for the future of social care for adults in England*. London: Department of Health

Godin, P. (ed.) (2006) *Risk and nursing practice*. Basingstoke: Palgrave Macmillan

Penhale, B. and Parker. J.(2008) *Working with vulnerable adults*. Abingdon: Routledge

Chapter 6

Values, Accountability and Responsibility

Key themes

In this chapter you will:

- examine those underlying values of the individual practitioner, and of the organisation under whose auspices care is provided, that have a direct impact on the quality of care that is received by the service user;

- reflect on care standards that are derived from these core values;

- reflect on the extent to which practitioners are responsible for the level of care that they provide;

- reflect on the accountability of practitioners.

INTRODUCTION

In the earlier chapters in this book we have explored and unpacked the values inherent in health and social care and have reflected on how these values can be integrated into practice. The values that underpin care interventions are probably one of the most significant determinants of the quality of the care that an individual receives, and understanding them is consequently of enormous importance. The values that are expressed by different groups in the care sector dictate the standards of care that are subsequently developed, and these are then reflected directly in the care that is provided to service users.

Quality of care provision is thus determined by values and by the standards that are derived from those values. These standards are monitored and audited to assess whether the agreed requirements have been met. If care provision is found to be wanting, practitioners may be asked to account for their actions, and the actions of others. In order to account for their actions practitioners need to understand both what they are doing and why they are doing it. This chapter will consider what it means to be responsible and accountable in a care role and will reflect on why understanding values is a crucial consideration in providing good, responsible and effective care.

It is probably safe to say that practitioners rarely overtly discuss their underpinning values with their individual clients directly, even though these values are the fundamental determinants of the kind of care that the care recipient will ultimately receive. Instead, values underpinning care provision are articulated on behalf of the care practitioner in a variety of different forms. These can be formal and legally binding expectations of values and standards of care, as expressed in codes of practice, such as the *Code of Practice for Social Care Workers* (GSCC, 2002), national occupational standards or national service frameworks, which formally articulate underpinning values and standards for care provision. Or they can be a more informal expression of values and intentions as articulated in vision statements and philosophies of care.

Reading activity

Conduct a search to see how many different expressions of standards you can find that are relevant to your work area. Were you aware of the promises that have been made about the service you will be providing? Do you feel adequately prepared to provide that service?

Examples of places to look may be: the Department of Health website, the General Social Care Council (GSCC) website, Skills for Health, Skills for Care and the websites of other relevant professional organisations and societies. You may also look in your workplace to see if there is a vision statement, expression of service standards or commitments or an expressed philosophy of care.

RESPONSIBILITY AND ACCOUNTABILITY IN PRACTICE

Providing care for others must be differentiated from work in other occupations. Care work cannot be viewed as 'just a job', in the way that working at the checkout in a supermarket could be viewed. Unlike customers in a supermarket, clients are often vulnerable and need to place their trust in another's hands. Unlike a supermarket, individuals in a care setting are inviting strangers to participate in the most private and intimate aspects of their lives. Also, unlike a supermarket, if service users do not like the service they receive they are frequently unable to take their business elsewhere. Care workers are in a very privileged, but also very responsible, position. It has been claimed that the way in which we treat the most vulnerable in society is a reflection of the values, ethics, compassion and standards of that society (Seedhouse, 1998). In order to protect the most vulnerable, and for society to fulfil its obligations to those that are most vulnerable, standards of practice are set. These standards are derived from the underlying beliefs and values about how we should treat our fellow humans.

When a practitioner provides care they enter into a 'contract' with a service user. This 'contract' imposes a special duty and responsibility on the care giver towards the person receiving care and requires the care giver to meet specified standards. If the care falls below expected standards the practitioner may be called upon to justify and account for their actions. What this means is that practitioners in care owe a greater duty and responsibility to their clients than do people in other service occupations.

Responsible and accountable

Being responsible means that certain expectations of behaviour are projected on to an individual when undertaking a particular role, and when these expectations are not met the individual who should have fulfilled the expectations can be called to account or, at worst, blamed for the failures. Different roles entail different responsibilities. As a parent I am responsible for the well-being, support and development of my children. As a teacher I may be responsible for meeting the learning needs of my students. As a care giver I am responsible for facilitating the health, well-being and, where possible, rehabilitation of those within my care. As a manager I am responsible for the overall policies and procedures of an organisation and, therefore, I may also share some of the responsibility for the actions of the people who work within that organisation. Different roles bring different levels of responsibility and these responsibilities need to be understood as an inevitable part of life. From a very early age we begin to acquire responsibility. However, although we must be mindful of our different responsibilities, it is also important to recognise the boundaries of these.

It is not until we reach the age of 18, when the law recognises us as adults, that we become fully responsible. However, although our parents may be ultimately legally responsible for us until we reach the age of maturity, it does not mean that the law condones irresponsible or criminal behaviour before this time. As soon as children can understand and make decisions they may share responsibility for their actions. As adults we are deemed to be sufficiently capable of making decisions for ourselves, by ourselves, and we can, therefore, be held legally and morally responsible for the actions and consequences that arise from those decisions and actions. When we are responsible we are also accountable. That means that we may be called upon to explain our actions (or failure to act) to someone who has the right to ask. It is very difficult to disassociate responsibility and accountability, except in those personal decisions that affect only me. I may be responsible for myself but I am not required to account to myself for my actions (although it could be argued that this is the process that occurs in truly, effective, reflective practice). As a general rule if we are responsible then we are also accountable to somebody.

To whom am I responsible and accountable?

The service user

When we enter into a care relationship with another person, as well as being responsible for ourselves we also take on some responsibility towards that person. This responsibility brings with it the requirement for particular standards of performance to be maintained. In the case of the care worker this responsibility is expressed in law as a 'duty of care'. The duty of care is owed to any person for whom you are caring in an occupational capacity. This duty applies to all activities undertaken by the care worker, whether it is complex surgery or simply assisting with washing an individual. This duty of care requires that any intervention undertaken by the care worker must be done to an 'appropriate standard'. It can be argued, however, that an appropriate standard is a very vague term. This is partly because the environment of care is constantly changing and partly because it would be impossible to articulate every element of care provision in every circumstance. Therefore, there has to be an element of interpretation in what the law means in relation to an 'appropriate standard'.

The law

The judgement of whether an action is appropriate or not is made by applying a common principle – i.e., practitioners will be judged by measuring their performance against the standard achieved by the 'ordinary, competent practitioner' undertaking that same role. That is to say, if your practice is called into question, you will be judged on the basis of the normal standards of behaviour expected of other practitioners in similar roles to yours. The key words in this judgement are 'ordinary' and 'competent'. Practitioners are not measured against the standard of the very best practitioner or against the latest techniques, unless these have become common practice, but are judged against generally acceptable practice. This standard has been set to recognise the fact that practitioners are human and that they cannot be expected to always deliver exemplary care at the forefront of the discipline. However, it also recognises that service users are entitled to generally acceptable care that at least meets minimum standards.

The other requirement of the law is that the practitioner must be 'competent' within their sphere of expertise and within the expectations of their role. It is, therefore, important that training and education have been provided to enable the practitioner to undertake the practices that they are required to do. It also means that practitioners must meet the minimum standards of safety and proficiency following any training that has been undertaken.

Ideas about acceptable and competent practice change as work practices develop. These developments are often the result of research and new evidence and this is what is meant by the term 'evidence-based practice'. In order to fulfil the requirement for evidence-based practice, the care practitioner is responsible for ensuring that their knowledge and practice are up to date. Not all practitioners are required to generate evidence, but they are required to be aware of evidence and base their practices upon it.

A duty of care, however, is not a licence to control others and make decisions for them about their care, decisions that they should be making for themselves (see Chapter 3 on autonomy). Neither is the duty of care a requirement to undertake roles outside of one's sphere of expertise and experience. It must be understood that my responsibility to a service user may require me to pass aspects of, or all of, their care on to someone more appropriate if the service user's needs are outside of my knowledge and experience. Knowing the limits of my ability, and the appropriate action to take, is an important aspect of responsibility.

Responsibility to the employer

As an employee I am responsible for ensuring that I understand, agree with and fulfil the employment obligations laid down in my contract of employment. This usually means that I am required to undertake a particular role and fulfil a contracted number of hours in that role. In addition, I will be required to ensure that I act in accordance with the policies and procedures of that organisation. Failure to adhere to policies may require me to account for my actions to a manager or to a disciplinary hearing. It should be remembered that, while the employer should make policies easily available to me, I am responsible for knowing and implementing the policies. As with other situations, ignorance is no defence.

Responsible for others

As practitioners become more senior they are likely to assume responsibility not only for their own actions but also for the actions of others. In the same way that practitioners owe a duty of care and responsibility to service users, so too do they owe a duty and responsibility to those fellow workers for whose care they are also responsible. Managers are responsible for ensuring that other practitioners are appropriately prepared and trained for the tasks that they are being asked to undertake and that they are properly supervised and supported while fulfilling their roles. The principle is that individuals should not be placed in situations in which they are out of their depth or where they may pose a threat to themselves or others. There are no hard-and-fast rules about what this means in practice and each situation and each individual must be assessed independently. Before tasks are delegated to others the manager must be reasonably confident that the task is within the individual's scope of competence. It is also important to note that even though an individual has received training in a particular task, it cannot necessarily be assumed that they will be competent at performing that task. If they have had little opportunity to practise the task, they may not be competent. Checking by asking the individual, or observing them undertake the task for the first time, is a responsible way of assuring oneself of their competence. From time to time things will not go as planned or as foreseen and this is an unfortunate fact of life. If an issue does arise, the manager as well as the care practitioner must be able to account for the actions and the decisions that they have made. That is, they must be able to explain what they did and why they did it.

Responsibility and the employer

The employer also has responsibilities in the care environment, both to the service users and to the care workers. The employer is responsible for ensuring that care provision can be conducted in a safe environment and that appropriate equipment is provided to undertake the job safely. The employer is also responsible for ensuring that the employees have access to appropriate training and development in order to perform their role. By virtue of the fact that the employer has employed the employee, the employer assumes vicarious (on your behalf) responsibility for the actions of that employee. If, therefore, an employee is negligent or causes harm to an individual in their care, the employer will be held responsible and accountable for that harm, alongside the employee; although it is usual for the employer to incur any financial compensation costs that are awarded as a result of that harm. However, the employee may be the subject of an internal disciplinary hearing or even a criminal prosecution if their actions are sufficiently serious.

Responsibility for the manner in which care is provided

While the practitioner has a legal responsibility to provide competent care (that is, they know what to do and can demonstrate that they are able to do it), most care practitioners will also have a responsibility to provide care in a particular manner. It is easy to teach someone to do a task competently. In fact, it has been demonstrated that other species such as monkeys can be taught to undertake tasks competently. However, the fact that a task has been performed is not sufficient. For the person receiving the care, the way the care is provided is of equal importance to the fact that care has been provided.

Discussion activity

Imagine that you are in hospital waiting to have surgery. You have spoken to the surgeon who was very knowledgeable and who told you all the technicalities of the operation. You also saw the anaesthetist who has explained her role. The nurse has explained that you will be unable to eat and drink prior to the surgery. You will be taken to the theatre at 11 o'clock and will return to the ward once you are sufficiently awake. They have all asked you whether you have understood what is going to happen. You have had your vital signs recorded, your blood taken for relevant tests and you have signed a consent form. You have been safely prepared for theatre and are aware of what to expect. In the middle of the night you wake up scared. You call the nurse who stands by you and repeats everything that you have been told during the day. Having finished, she walks away to attend to someone else.

1. Do you think that the nurse has provided competent care?
2. What else could the nurse have done to provide you with better care?

I think it is clear that the professionals providing the care in this case have done that which is technically required of them in relation to competent care. However, as a service user, I would feel let down if this had happened to me. Care that is only based on competence ceases to acknowledge the importance of the other essential component, the values base of care. The nurse could have acted differently. She could have sat down and held the individual's hand and acknowledged their right to be afraid. She may have let the service user talk about their fears. She may even have sought to provide evidence that their fears were likely to be unfounded. She may have done nothing more than sit with them and provided support. However, by acknowledging how the individual feels and taking their feelings seriously, I believe the service user would have felt valued. Their fears about the forthcoming surgery may not be any less after the interaction, particularly as the nurse could not change the fact that the individual was still going to endure surgery, but the client may have a much more positive view of their experience. That human demonstration of empathy may make a significant difference to how the individual approaches their surgery. Competence is, of course, a very important aspect of care provision, but the inclusion of compassion and the influence of the care value-base lift the care provided from good care to that which is exceptional and memorable.

PROFESSIONAL ACCOUNTABILITY AND CODES OF PRACTICE

The values that are evident in care are often not legal responsibilities but 'professional' responsibilities. These values are articulated in codes of practice. These codes set out the standards and expectations of different groups of practitioners and seek to articulate the specific beliefs and practices that the public can expect when in contact with that group. When we fail to meet the value standards of our 'professional' group, individuals have a right to report us to the organisations that regulate practice.

Codes of practice provide practitioners with broad principles to guide their actions and behaviours. However, they cannot be used as a rulebook to tell practitioners what to do in every situation. Although codes of practice have an important role in guiding practitioner behaviours, they have also been criticised because of the ambiguity that they can create when two or more of the guiding principles expressed in the codes conflict (Wainwright and Pattison, 2004).

Discussion activity

With a colleague, reflect on the GSCC *Code of Practice for Social Care Workers* (GSCC, 2002) and try to identify any conflicting principles. Discuss what practitioners can do when faced with apparently conflicting guiding principles.

If a regulatory body is alerted that an individual has breached the code of practice, an investigation will occur and the practitioner may be called to account for their actions at a hearing. Such a hearing carries no weight in law but may adversely impact on the individual's specific role or rights to work in that kind of employment. If the complaint is sufficiently serious it could result in legal prosecution as well. For example, if a care worker is accused of hitting someone in their care they would be in breach of the code of practice but also would be at risk of prosecution for assault. In care practice we have a responsibility to and for service users, to our employers to ensure that we fulfil the requirements of our role, to the law, and we may also have a responsibility to a regulatory body. Wherever it can be demonstrated that we have a responsibility we may be called to account for our actions in relation to that responsibility. That is we may be asked to justify what we have done and why we have done it.

When called to account, in any of the circumstances identified above, there are several ways that this account can be given. This is sometimes in person at an interview or by giving formal evidence. However, this could be in other forms such as production of care records or a formal written statement of events. Accurate record keeping is therefore of vital importance in evidencing care provision and underlying values.

MAINTAINING RECORDS

The maintenance of accurate and contemporary records plays an important role in ensuring consistent, planned care and the appropriate review and assessment of care. However, records may also be used to account for your practice. In spite of the important role that record keeping plays in care provision, it is often seen as a burdensome chore and it is well documented that it is an activity that is done badly (Dimond, 2005; Reid, 2006). Reviews of records in social care (Trevithick, 2005) have criticised records for:

- failing to record baseline information;
- failure to note deterioration or improvement of condition;
- failure to record decisions or conversations;
- failure to link information together;
- failure to provide indications of future care and intervention.

Looking at this list, one could be forgiven for wondering what role records are fulfilling. Perhaps it is because records are seen as an irksome activity that gets in the way of the real job of caring that they are so badly kept. However, it cannot be stressed too much that accurate and careful record keeping is for the good and protection of the care worker as well as the service user.

Writing activity

Look at this list of the purposes of records and tick the ones you think are relevant:

- a legal requirement;
- as a story about the client's care;
- as a means of communication between different practitioners;

- a report to document improvements, deteriorations, deviations from plans;
- a record for goals and action plans;
- as a means of documenting a client's express wishes;
- as a means of ensuring consistency of care;
- as a legal record of care and the treatment provided;
- to record interactions with clients and family;
- to protect the practitioner from claims that they did not provide good care;
- as a historical record.

Hopefully you ticked all, or nearly all, of the above as they all have a role to play in the maintenance of records.

There is a tension in record keeping between recording sufficient accurate information and maintaining a succinct and manageable record. Coulshed and Orme (1998) state that records should keep an account of: 'significant facts, evidence, feelings, decisions, action taken, planned action and when actions should be monitored and reviewed'. One could add: tests undertaken; results received and significant conversations with clients or relevant others. Ensuring the accuracy of information in records is essential. Practitioners should avoid recording value judgements and hearsay and should avoid statements that do not convey any useful information such as, for example, 'usual care given' or 'needs assistance with walking'. If a practitioner was asked at a later date to account for what that meant specifically, they would probably be unable to remember the specifics of that particular person's care. It is much better to briefly note what was actually done for the individual and what specific assistance is needed. It is a salutary lesson to stop and think 'if I am asked about this in five years' time in a court of law, will I know what I meant?' 'Will there be enough information in my records to help me remember the specific care that was given to that particular person and the reasons for the care that was provided?'

An increasingly common method of validating records is, where possible, to do this in partnership with service users. As a nurse it often used to frustrate me to read in the notes the person had 'slept well' only to be told by the patient, 'I had such a bad night, nurse'. Service users are keen to be involved in their care and, while it may take more time, it is likely to improve the accuracy of the records written.

Statements as an account of practice

Formal statements may be used as a legal document to assess what happened at an event or to make a judgement about the quality and circumstances of someone's care. Statements should be used as a means of recording a factual account of events to the best of your knowledge. Detail is important, but only relevant detail. Statements should not be used as an opportunity to suggest who else could be to blame or to pass opinions on others' behaviours and actions. Neither are they an opportunity to write a story.

Writing activity

1. Read the statement in Figure 6.1 and underline the facts of the case in one colour. Then, in another colour, underline anything that you think is hearsay or assumption or irrelevant material.
2. Rewrite the statement as a factual account of events.
3. Reflect on the values and actions of the care assistant expressed in this statement and think about how the values expressed influenced the unfortunate outcome of the situation. How should the care assistant have acted?

A medication error

Saturday 24 May 2007. The nurse, Julie Brown, came on duty as usual at 7.45, even though she was due on duty at 7.30. I think she had difficulty getting out of bed, but nobody seemed to bother, it's not fair, everyone else has to get to the ward on time. Anyway, because she is late it always made it late when medicines are given out and I expect that on this morning she had to rush to get things done. Nurse Brown gave the medicines out as usual and then we, the care assistants, had to do the washes. We always have to do the boring jobs. On this morning I was asked to help Florence with her wash. My heart sank. I find her difficult to cope with because she always asks questions about everything you do. When I got there she asked me, if the water was hot? and had I got her clean clothes? She didn't want the green cardigan I had got out, but wanted me to change it for the red one, I've been looking after her long enough, I know what she likes. She is lucky that anyone does anything for her! Half way through the wash she asked me why Nurse Brown had given her different pills today. I told her that the nurse knows what she is doing and that the doctor had probably changed her prescription. I asked if she had taken her pills, but she said that she hadn't because she did not know what they were. I said that they must be right if the nurse had given them to her and I stood by her while she took them. Later on the nurse called me into the office and said that Florence had been given the wrong pills and that I had to write a statement. It's not my fault that she took the wrong pills. I am not responsible for giving patients their pills. That nurse should have checked more carefully.

Figure 6.1 Medication error

The statement has been used by the care worker as a platform to complain about her role, complain about a patient and complain about her colleagues and their actions, even though all of this is opinion and outside the responsibilities of her role. She has recounted the actual facts of the situation but these are hidden among lots of subjective statements and conjecture. She attempts to push the responsibility of her actions on to the nurse, who may have made an initial error in giving the wrong tablets, but the error was then compounded by the care worker who overrode the concerns of the patient. The statement is a clear expression of the care worker's values. She fails to respect service users, she clearly sees individual care as burdensome and she abuses her position as a care worker to control the actions of those in her care. However, while assuming a position of power in relation to the patient, she is reluctant to assume that responsibility when called to account and fails to recognise her own responsibility in relation to the drug error.

CONCLUSION

Care workers are required to make endless decisions in their day-to-day work. The decisions they face are often not easy and there are frequently no absolute rules about how to act. Care work is a responsible activity and, in fulfilling that responsibility, care workers need to be guided by core care values, codes of practice and standards of care, all of which articulate the expectations that should be met. It is also a fact that care workers will be called to account for what they have done and, at times, for what they have failed to do. Responsibility and accountability are, of necessity, indivisible.

Accountability is an essential component of the protection of the public. However, accountability serves another purpose too. It is a mechanism through which practice can be monitored, reflected upon and, where necessary, improvements can be made. Care workers are responsible to those in their care, their employers and sometimes their regulatory body. They are required by law to fulfil their duty of care to service users and their carers. Care workers may be called to account for their actions informally or formally, either in person or through written records or formal statements.

Good record keeping is essential in ensuring that the practitioner is able to communicate effectively to others and to provide evidence that will assist the practitioner to recollect actual care provided and account for their actions.

The essential component of good quality care is the need to ground all care within the care value base and to understand that how we do something is just as important as what we do. If values remain at the heart of practice then care will not only be competent but will also be respectful, caring and compassionate, and responsibility and accountability will not be such frightening concepts.

SUMMARY OF KEY POINTS

- This chapter has identified that care work requires practitioners to be responsible for both their actions and their failures to act when they should have done. It also identifies that when you assume responsibilities you may be called to account if these responsibilities are not met.

- An important source of your account of care is contained within records written by care workers. These records may be accessed years after the care event to explore care provision. This chapter has identified the imperative of maintaining current, accurate, factual and concise records.

FURTHER READING

Audit Commission (1995) *Setting the records straight*. London: Audit Commission

HSC annual report. London: Health Service Commissioner

Chapter 7

Conclusion – Value-based Reflection

THE ROLE OF VALUES

In this book we have focused on the key values that we consider to be an essential component of good care practice. As has been discussed, caring has a qualitative dimension and demands more from the practitioner than simply performing a task. This dimension says something about the way in which care should be carried out. The chapters in this book have explored the key values that define the care standards that individual practitioners should observe in their activities and relationships with service users. Many of the individuals in receipt of care, at some time, are likely also to experience vulnerability; either by virtue of illness, age, disability, pain or loss of confidence. As has been claimed earlier in the book, the way a society treats its most vulnerable is a measure of the moral character of that society (Seedhouse, 1998). We have therefore claimed in this book that values are an essential component of good care practice.

The merit of a set of articulated values has been discussed elsewhere in the book but, in summary, values:

- set universally acceptable standards of behaviour;
- provide a guide for practitioners to provide and reflect on care;
- provide a benchmark for others to judge standards of care.

However, it should be noted that, while agreed values provide a guide for practitioner behaviour, they are not a set of rules. At times your values will conflict with each other and, sometimes, they will conflict with the service users', or other practitioners', beliefs or judgements. This book explores values in care and discusses the origins and reasons for the selection of these values and their application to care practice. The activities in this book have been devised to enable you to explore your own values and practice and to reflect on these in the light of the expressed values under-pinning care practice. Think about what you have learned about yourself and about others from participating in the activities in this book. It is true to say that you will face value-based challenges for as long as you practise. In fact, it would be worrying if you did not, as this might indicate that your practice was routinised and unresponsive to individual needs and situations. This chapter will briefly summarise the values that have been addressed in this book, before looking to the future and asking how you can ensure that values are fully integrated into your care practice.

Rights, equality and anti-discriminatory practice

The chapter on rights, equality and anti-discriminatory practice is important in setting the context for much of the care practice in today's health and care system. The language of rights or entitlements provides legitimacy for individuals to seek the kind of care that they need or desire. Charters of rights are published by different groups to articulate their expectations and to provide a vehicle for challenging care when these expectations are not met. Generally, the rights that are articulated and claimed, particularly in the care context, are claims on another person or authority to provide the thing claimed. This is often the problem with a purely rights-based approach. Such an approach does not really help the practitioner who is faced by a rights claim but who may not have the resources available to meet the claim. Nor does this approach to care help the practitioner to adjudicate between competing claims. For example, if there were two people in equal need of a wheelchair, but only one wheelchair, how would the practitioner decide whose right it is to have their need met? However, in spite of these obvious difficulties, the publication and assertion of rights are very useful in both articulating entitlements and expectations, and for providing a vehicle through which care shortcomings can be challenged.

Rights rhetoric has also been the most influential factor in ensuring that more equal and fair treatment is available for those who have been unable to make their voice heard in other ways. Legislation to address issues around equality and various types of discrimination has been an essential component in raising awareness and providing fairer opportunities for those in marginalised and discriminated groups. It is a shameful fact that discriminatory behaviour is still alive and well and is still widely perpetrated in the care environment. A focus on rights means that this is gradually improving and provides a platform to challenge and, where appropriate, prosecute anyone who persists in discriminatory behaviour.

Respect, dignity and autonomy

It is, perhaps, a sad reflection on the way that others are treated that a rights rhetoric is necessary. If all people were afforded the respect that they were due, by virtue of being a person, irrespective of age, sex, ability, colour or race, there should be no need to resort to claims for rights. The chapters on respect, dignity and autonomy demonstrate that respect is a fundamental value in care practice. Understanding respect for persons is a core value and, if this is properly understood and integrated into care, many of the other values will flow from it. Respect for persons in care facilitates the partnership philosophy of care that promotes dignity for clients even in situations of great dependence.

Being respected, having our views taken seriously, being able to express our individuality, being able to make, and act on, our own decisions and choices, and being able to devise our own goals, are very prized features of our everyday lives. It is these things that give us a sense of worth and a sense of self. It follows then that, if these things are important to us, they are also of equal importance to those for whom we provide care. The chapters on respect, dignity and autonomy explored the notion and extent of respect and examined the duties of the care practitioner in ensuring that these values underpin practice. The activities in these chapters provided you with an opportunity to examine your own approach to care and to think about strategies that would enable you to enhance respect and dignity and provide opportunities to support those in your care to be autonomous.

Trust, confidentiality and truth-telling

This chapter identified that all caring and therapeutic relationships need to be established on the foundation of trust. Care recipients trust practitioners to act in their best interests, to be knowledgeable, to be caring in their approach and to do them no harm. Practitioners trust clients to be honest and to work in partnership with them. The notion of trust is important in any relationship. However, it is even more important in the care relationship where the service user puts themselves in another's hands, often a complete stranger, and then allows them access to the most private and intimate aspects of their lives, both physical and emotional. In such situations the practitioner is very privileged and carries a huge responsibility to respect that trust placed in them and to take the responsibility of the caring role very seriously.

In order to care effectively it is also frequently necessary to know information about others to which one is not normally privy. In view of this, the care practitioner is trusted, through the principle of confidentiality, to keep safe the information they are entrusted with. This is not always an easy and clear-cut activity and the appropriate sharing of information can be very confusing and challenging. The section on confidentiality provided you with an opportunity to explore the nature, limits and potential exceptions to the rule of confidentiality. In addition, this chapter explored the concept of truth and the notion of truth-telling as a fundamental feature of trust in the care relationship.

Protection from harm and promoting independence

At times a service user cannot or does not want to be autonomous, or sometimes expectations are placed on us by others which suggest that keeping a client safe and protecting them from harm are in the client's best interests. While protection from harm and a client's best interests are often at opposite ends of the spectrum, it is not true that they always are so. The chapter on protection from harm and promoting independence recognised the responsibility that practitioners have in protecting those in their care from harm. However, the chapter tried to do this from the 'respect for persons' perspective. In contemporary care, protection from harm and risk management have become dominant considerations, and are frequently the motivating factor for care decisions. This chapter argued that, although these are obviously important, they cannot be the only considerations on which care is based. While we must act in the client's best interests it might be argued that best interests are not always served by being overly protective.

The chapter argued that risk is an essential, and often enjoyable, feature of all our lives. Taking risks can enhance our lives. Even when risk taking goes wrong we gain valuable learning and this contributes to our personal development. The tension for the care practitioner is to try to establish what risks are acceptable and what responsibilities they hold towards those in their care in terms of protecting them from harm. The chapter provided a model for managed risk taking, which provides the practitioner with a framework for considering risks, in discussion, where possible, with the service user and other relevant parties, and provides practitioners with evidence of that consideration.

Values, accountability and responsibility

The final chapter in the book explored the relationship between values and the notions of accountability and responsibility. This chapter identified that if you engage in a care interaction with another you are responsible for ensuring your capability to undertake care and you are also responsible for the standard of your care provision. You are also accountable for your actions and you may be asked to explain your actions to anyone who has a right to ask; this could be the client, the employer, a professional or regulatory body, or the law. It is therefore important to understand what you are doing and why you are doing it, and not to undertake activities that are beyond the scope of your capability. Standards of care and codes of practice have been devised to provide a guide for practitioners and protection for clients. It is your responsibility to be aware of the standards and codes that relate to your own area of practice and to reflect on your practice in the light of these expectations.

Another important aspect of accountability is the records that are kept in respect of care provided. Records should provide evidence of actual care given. It is important that they are factual, informative and clear; they should note any changes in the service user's condition or situation and any significant conversation with that individual, their relatives or other practitioners. Records should not contain judgemental statements, hearsay or vague statements. Records provide a platform from which other practitioners can plan further care. Records also enable practitioners to assess a service user's progress or deterioration. If you are ever called to account for your actions, your records will be used to provide evidence of the care you provided.

WHERE TO NEXT?

This book has argued that understanding and integrating core values into care practice is an essential component of good care. So now you have read the book and explored these key values, what do you do with the information and how do you know that you have been successful in integrating values into your practice?

Reading a book on values will not necessarily provide you with a prescription to solve the next difficult situation that you encounter in practice. This book provides you with knowledge about why a value is important, what the tensions might be in adopting a value, and provides you with some examples of how values can be integrated into your practice. The next step is for you to take. Nobody's practice will ever change or improve if they always do what they have always done, in the way that they have always done it.

Value-led reflection

It is our belief that concentrating on values, that is to say understanding how and why you do what you do, is the most important means of improving your practice. We recommend that 'value-led reflection' is an important skill to learn. Reflective practice is well accepted in the care environment and there are a number of different models that can be used such as, for example, Kolb (1984) and Rolfe (2001). Reflective practice requires a practitioner to think about their practice and examine what they do in the light of theory. In addition, it offers the opportunity to change their practice or to justify to themselves and others that they have acted appropriately. 'Value-led reflection' uses the same skills but requires the practitioner to use values as the focus for their reflection.

Reflecting on values provides you with an opportunity to analyse your own value base and examine the care you currently provide in the light of the care you would like to provide. In addition, value-led reflection helps you to think through a rationale for care and to think about strategies to overcome barriers to providing value-led care. Reflective practice is often interpreted as reflecting on critical or dramatic incidents in order to see if this could have been addressed differently. We suggest that value-led reflection is most valuable when it is used to explore and analyse aspects of everyday care; things that become so routine and second nature to the practitioner that they are no longer consciously aware of how or why they do them in the way that they do. Hopefully, by learning to engage in value-led reflection, you will start to see what you do with new eyes, what Schön identifies as 'extraordinarily re-experiencing the ordinary' (Schön, 1987, p.93).

As discussed previously, there is no magic formula that outlines exactly how you must interact and provide care. How you do it will not necessarily mirror how a colleague may undertake the same activity. What is important is that your approach reflects your values and the needs, expectations and values of the care recipient and, in addition, that you can draw on a framework that enables you to account to others for your actions.

Value-led reflection does not need to be done as an isolated activity. The exercise is just as valuable when undertaken in a group. The added advantage is that when there are differences of understanding you have an opportunity to explore others' beliefs, values and interpretations and you will develop a better understanding of the factors that impact on your and others' practice. Once you are confident about the dominant values that guide your own personal practice you may choose to share this with those in your care. This is particularly helpful in preventing frustrations that may result from differences in expectations. If the service user is under the impression that you, as the practitioner, will do everything for them, they will feel cheated and let down if your principal value is to facilitate independence.

The following is a series of statements that you can reflect upon to help you to engage in value-led reflection, and to help you identify your preferred personal values.

- You must answer honestly.
- They are not easy questions and most need in-depth consideration.
- When you have answered the questions you need to revisit them and ask yourself if these answers reflect the way that you would like to practise.

Reflection

What values underpin my practice?

1. I always treat all clients equally, irrespective of age, sex, race, disability, or condition.

Strongly agree	Agree	Disagree	Strongly disagree

2. Some clients are difficult to care for.

Strongly agree	Agree	Disagree	Strongly disagree

3. Ensuring that a client's choices are always met is very important to me.

Strongly agree	Agree	Disagree	Strongly disagree

4. Clients' choices should be overridden if an alternative course of action is in their best interests.

Strongly agree	Agree	Disagree	Strongly disagree

5. Practitioners often know what is in their client's best interests.

Strongly agree	Agree	Disagree	Strongly disagree

6. Only clients know what is in their best interests.

Strongly agree	Agree	Disagree	Strongly disagree

7. It is my responsibility to ensure that clients do not come to any harm.

Strongly agree	Agree	Disagree	Strongly disagree

8. Clients have the right to engage in activities, even when it has been identified that they might pose a risk.

Strongly agree	Agree	Disagree	Strongly disagree

9. All clients are entitled to have their rights respected.

Strongly agree	Agree	Disagree	Strongly disagree

10. Sometimes rights need to be balanced against the needs or rights of others.

Strongly agree	Agree	Disagree	Strongly disagree

Statements that you have strongly agreed or agreed with will demonstrate what your preferred approach to care is. This may veer towards a care approach that favours promoting autonomy and independence, or you may favour an approach that focuses more on support and protection. Neither approach is wrong. Knowing your starting place is very important.

The next set of questions you need to ask yourself are:

- Am I happy with this approach to care?
- Is this the kind of care I feel is appropriate?
- Is this the kind of care I would like to receive?

Think through some reasons why you have answered in the way that you have. This is a way of checking out the validity of your claims. Once you have established what your core values are, answer the following questions:

- Can I effectively integrate my core values into my practice?
- If not, what is stopping me?

Try to think of some examples from practice that illustrate when values have been effectively integrated into your practice, and then some examples of when you have had to compromise on your values. In these examples try to think what the barriers were. In view of the fact that a care relationship needs to encompass more than just the practitioner's views and beliefs, answer the following questions (and provide examples):

- What role do clients have in determining the care that they receive?
- Are you happy with this balance?

Value-led reflection is only as good as the action that it leads us to. Therefore it is necessary to take reflection on from 'a looking back' exercise to 'a looking forward' exercise.

- Is there anything that I should do differently in respect of the care that I provide? (Think about specific examples.)
- Are there any different strategies that I can use to get round some of the barriers?
- Do I need any help to address these issues? If so, what would that help be?
- Is there anything about the care that others around me provide that I am uncomfortable about?

What strategies could I use to address discomfort about others' practices?

If you have answered 'yes' to the final question it shows that you are using values to look at the wider context of care and your responsibilities as a practitioner. This is probably the most difficult area to work on, particularly if you are a junior member of a team. However, if you are feeling uncomfortable about another's practice it probably means that it would benefit from some exploration. In such a situation, there are a number of strategies available to you depending on the severity of your discomfort. Here are just a few possible ways of raising awareness of others' practices. However, please remember that, if these are serious concerns, you are accountable for what you see and know so you are responsible for making these concerns known to the appropriate manager or authority.

- You could adopt a genuinely interested stance and ask why someone does something in a particular way.
- You could ask another person if a particular action is acceptable practice or not (remember to maintain confidentiality).
- You could ask team members to engage in some shared reflective activities.
- You could look for some evidence that suggests a particular practice is unacceptable and discuss it with the practitioner concerned.
- You could challenge the practitioner directly.
- You may feel the need to report your concerns to someone in a position of authority.

There is rarely a clear-cut answer to the question: 'which strategy should I use?' Only you know your individual situation and circumstances. In addition, you need to consider the risks involved in engaging in any of the above strategies, as well as the risks of doing nothing. Do not forget that risks often pay off and have a positive outcome.

The purpose of value-led reflection is to help you to explore what kind of practitioner you want to be. It will help you to think about your practice in order to identify things that you can change in order to be more like the practitioner you want to be. Value-led reflection is not a once-only activity. It is a tool to be used again and again to check if you have developed bad habits or less good practice. Value-led reflection can also be used to help you decide what to do when you encounter new situations in care. Ultimately it is hoped that it will improve practice. Values are at the core of good practice. If you invest time reflecting on your values and the ways in which they impact on your care, and you try to adapt your care where possible in the light of this reflection, it is likely that your care will be improved, bringing greater satisfaction to you and the care recipient.

FURTHER READING

Ghaye, T. (2000) *Reflection: principles and practice for health care professionals.* Dinton: Quay Books

Johns, C. (2004) *Becoming a reflective practitioner.* Oxford: Blackwell

Tate, S. and Sills, M. (2006) *The development of critical reflection in the health professions.* London: HEA

References

Alaszewski, A., Harrison, L. and Manthorpe, J. (eds) (1998) *Risk, health and welfare*. Buckingham: Open University Press

Alderson, P. (2002) 'Young Children's Health Care Rights and Consent', in Franklin, B. (ed.) *The new handbook of children's rights. Comparative policy and practice*. London: Routledge

Alderson, P. (2000) *Young children's rights, exploring beliefs, principles and practice*. London: Jessica Kingsley

Alderson, P. and Montgomery, J. (1996) *Health care choices: making decisions with children*. London: Institute for Public Policy Research

Almond, B. (1991) 'Rights', in Singer, P. (ed.) (1993) *A companion to ethics*. Oxford: Blackwell Publishing

Allport, G. (1954) *The nature of prejudice*. Boston: Beacon Press

Audit Commission (2004) *Older people – independence and well-being: the challenge for public services*. London: Audit Commission

Baier, A. (1986) 'Trust and antitrust'. *Ethics*, 96, 231–60

Banks, S. (2001) *Ethics and values in social work*. 2nd ed. Houndmills, Basingstoke: Palgrave MacMillan

Banks, S. (2004) *Ethics, accountability and the social professions*. Houndmills, Basingstoke: Palgrave MacMillan

Banks, S. (2006) *Ethics and values in social work*. 3rd ed. Houndmills, Basingstoke: Palgrave

Beach, M.C., Duggan, P.S., Cassel, C.K. and Geller, G. (2007) 'What does "respect" mean? Exploring the moral obligation of health professionals to respect patients.' *Journal of Society of General Internal Medicine*, 22: 692—5

Beauchamp, T. and Childress, J.(2001) *Principles of biomedical ethics*. 5th ed. New York: Oxford University Press

Beck, U. (1992) *Risk society*. London: UCL Press

Blakemore, K. (2003) *Social policy. An introduction*. Buckingham: Open University Press

Boore, J.R.P.(1978) *Prescription for recovery: the effect of pre-operative preparation of surgical patients on post-operative stress, recovery and infection*. London: Royal College of Nursing

Brazier, M. and Lobjoit, M (1991) *Protecting the vulnerable. Autonomy and consent in health care*. London: Routledge

British Medical Association (2005) Confidentiality as part of the bigger picture. A discussion paper from the BMA. Available at **www.bma.org.uk/ap.nsf/Content/Con fidentialityBiggerPicture** (accessed 16 November 2007)

British Medical Association (2007) *Consent tool kit*. 3rd ed. London: BMA

Butterworth, C. (2005) 'Ongoing consent to care for older people in care homes.' *Nursing Standard*, 19 (20): 40–5

Christman, J. (2003) Autonomy in moral and political philosophy. *Stanford Encyclopedia of Philosophy* at **plato.stanford.edu/entries/autonomy-moral/** (accessed 30 June 2007)

College of Occupational Therapists (2005) *College of Occupational Therapists Code of Ethics and Professional Conduct*. London: COT

Commission for Racial Equality (2006) Evidence presented in a speech by Trevor Phillips, Chair of the Commission for Racial Equality

Coulshed, V. and Orme, J. (1998) *Social work practice: an introduction.* 3rd ed. Basingstoke: MacMillan BASW

Darwall, S. (1977) 'Two kinds of respect.' *Ethics*, 88: 36–49; reprinted in R.S. Dillon (ed.) *Dignity, character, and self-respect*, New York: Routledge, 1995

Denney, D. (2005) *Risk and society*. London: Sage Publications

Department for Constitutional Affairs (DCA) (2005) *Mental Capacity Act 2005. Summary* at **www.dca.gov.uk/legal-policy/mental-capacity/mca-summary.pdf** (accessed 14 February 2007)

Department for Constitutional Affairs (2007) *Mental Capacity Act 2005. Code of Practice*. Crown Copyright. London: The Stationery Office

Department for Education and Skills (2005) *Common core of skills and knowledge for the children's workforce*. Nottingham: DfES Publications

Department of Health (2000) NHS Plan. London: Department of Health

Department of Health (2001a) *National service framework for older people*. London: The Stationery Office

Department of Health (2001b) *Valuing people: a new strategy for learning disability for the 21st century*. London: The Stationery Office

Department of Health (2003a) *Essence of care. Patient-focused benchmarks for clinical governance. Guidance and Benchmarks*. April 2003. NHS Modernisation Agency

Department of Health (2003b) *NHS Code of Practice for confidentiality*. London: The Stationery Office

Department of Health (2004a) *Choosing health: making healthy choices easier*. London: The Stationery Office

Department of Health (2004b) *Seeking consent: working with older people*. London: The Stationery Office

Department of Health (2005a) Human Rights Case Studies **www.dh.gov.uk/PolicyAnd Guidance/EqualityAndHumanRights/** (accessed November 2005)

Department of Health (2005b) *Independence, well-being and choice: Our vision for the future of social care for adults in England*. London: The Stationery Office

Department of Health (2005c) *Research Governance Framework for Health and Social Care*. London: The Stationery Office

Department of Health (2006) *Our health, our care, our say: a new direction for community services*. London: The Stationery Office

Department of Health (2007) *Capabilities for inclusive practice*. August 2007. London: CSIP/DH

Dillon, R.S. (2007) 'Respect'. *Stanford Encyclopedia of Philosophy* at **plato.stanford.edu/ entries/respect/#ConRes** (accessed 14 June 2007)

Dillon, R.S. (1992) 'Respect and care: toward moral integration.' *Canadian Journal of Philosophy*, 22: 105–32

Dimond, B. (2004) *Legal aspects of nursing*. 4th ed. London: Longman

Dimond, B. (2005) 'Exploring common deficiencies that occur in record keeping.' *British Journal of Nursing*, 14(10): 568–70

Disabilities Rights Commission (2006) *Formal investigation into health inequalities – equal treatment: closing the gap*. London: DRC

Donnelly, E. and Neville, l. (2008) *Health and Social Care Knowledge and Skills: Communication and Interpersonal Skills*. Exeter: Reflect Press Ltd.

Downie, R.S. and Calman, K.C. (1994) *Healthy respect. Ethics in health care*. 2nd ed. Oxford: Oxford University Press

Doyal, L. and Gough, I. (1991) *A theory of human need*, Basingstoke: Macmillan

Dworkin, G. (1988) *The theory and practice of autonomy.* New York: Cambridge University Press

Fullbrook, S. (2007) The physical restraint of patients: can it ever be justified? *British Journal of Healthcare Assistants,* 1 (1): 41–2

Furedi, F. (1997) *Culture of fear: risk-taking and the morality of low expectation. Department of Health (2005a) Human Rights Case Studies* **www.dh.gov.uk/PolicyAnd Guidance/EqualityAndHumanRights/** (accessed November 2005). London: Cassell

Gale, T., Hawley, J. and Sivakumaran, T. (2003) 'Do mental health professionals really understand probability? Implications for risk assessment and evidence-based practice'. *Journal of Mental Health,*12(4):, 417–30

Garrett, T.M., Baillie, H.W. and Garrett, R.M. (2001) *Health care ethics: principles and problems.* 4th ed. Englewood Cliffs, N.J.: Prentice Hall

General Social Care Council (2002) *Code of Practice for Social Care Workers.* London: GSCC

Gilchrist, A. (1992) 'The revolution of everyday life revisited: towards an anti-discriminatory praxis for community work.' *Social Action,* 1(1): 22–8

Gillon, R. (1986) *Philosophical medical ethics.* Chichester: John Wiley & Sons

Handy, C.B. (1997) *Understanding organizations.* 4th ed. London: Penguin Business

Harris, J. (ed.) (2001) *Bioethics.* Oxford: Oxford University Press.

Harris, J. (1985) *The value of life. An introduction to medical ethics.* London: Routledge

Hayward, J. (1975) *Information – a prescription against pain.* London: Royal College of Nursing

Healthcare Commission (2007) *Inpatients: The views of hospital inpatients in England. Key Findings from the 2006 Survey.* London: Commission for Healthcare Audit and Inspection, at **www.healthcarecommission.org.uk/_db/_documents/Inpatient_survey_ briefing_note.pdf** (accessed 22 July 2007)

Help the Aged (2005) *Rights at risk – older people and human rights.* London: Help the Aged

Help the Aged (2007) 'Too old: older people's accounts of discrimination, exclusion and rejection.' *Report on Age Discrimination (RoAD) Research Project.* London: Help the Aged

Hendrick, J. (2004) *Law and ethics. Foundations in nursing and health care.* Cheltenham: Nelson Thornes

Hill, T. (1998) 'Respect for persons', in Craig, E. (ed.) *Routledge Encyclopaedia of Philosophy.* **www.rep.routledge.com/article/LO84SECT1** (accessed 10 February 2004)

Hupcey, J.E. and Miller, J. (2006) 'Community dwelling adults' perception of interpersonal trust vs trust in health care providers.' *Journal of Clinical Nursing,*15: 1132–39

Jackson, E. (2006) *Medical law. Text, cases and materials.* Oxford: Oxford University Press

Joffe, H. (2003) 'Risk: from perception to representation.' *British Journal of Social Psychology,* 42: 55–73

Jones, C. (2003) 'The utilitarian argument for medical confidentiality: a pilot study of patients' views.' *Journal of Medical Ethics,* 29: 348–52

Karakowsky, I. and Elangovan, A. (2001) 'Risky decision making in mixed gender teams. Whose tolerance counts?' *Small Group Research,* 32(1): 94–111

Kemshall, H. and Pritchard, J. (eds) (1996) *Good practice in risk assessment and risk management.* Vol. 1. London: Jessica Kingsley

Kolb, D. (1984) *Experiential learning: experience as the source of learning and development.* London: Prentice-Hall

Lockwood, M. (1985) *Moral dilemmas in modern medicine.* Oxford: Oxford University Press

Lupton, D. (1999) *Risk.* London: Routledge

Mason, J.K., Laurie, G.T. and Aziz, M. (2005) *Mason and McCall Smith's law and medical ethics.* Oxford: Oxford University Press

McLeod, C. (2006) 'Trust', in *Stanford Encyclopedia of Philosophy* at **http://plato.stanford. edu/entries/trust/** (accessed 10 November 2007)

Nursing and Midwifery Council (2004) *The NMC Code of Professional Conduct: standards for conduct, performance and ethics* at **www.nmc-uk.org/nmc/main/public ations/TheNMCcodeofprofessionalconduct.doc** (accessed 15 February 2005)

Nursing and Midwifery Council (2006) *The NMC Position Statement on the covert administration of medicines – Disguising medicine in food and drink.* Last updated March 2006 at **www.nmc-uk.org/aFrameDisplay.aspx?DocumentID=3397** (accessed 23 November 2007) or in their A-Z Advice at **www.nmc-uk.org/aSection.aspx?Section ID=11#sectionD** (accessed 23 November 2007)

O'Neill, O. (2002a) *A question of trust.* The BBC Reith Lectures 2002. Cambridge: Cambridge University Press, or available as transcripts at **www.bbc.co.uk/radio4/ reith2002/lectures.shtml** (accessed 26 October 2007)

O'Neill, O. (2002b) *A question of trust. Spreading suspicion.* Reith Lectures 2002. Lecture 1. BBC Radio 4, transcript at **www.bbc.co.uk/radio4/reith2002/lectures.shtml** (accessed 26 October 2007)

O'Neill, O. (2002c) *A question of trust. Trust and terror.* Reith Lectures 2002. Lecture 2, BBC Radio 4, transcript at **www.bbc.co.uk/radio4/reith2002/lectures.shtml** (accessed 26 October 2007)

O'Neill, O. (2002d) *A question of trust. Trust and transparency.* Reith Lectures 2002. Lecture 4. BBC Radio 4, transcript at **www.bbc.co.uk/radio4/reith2002/lect ures.shtml** (accessed 26 October 2007)

O'Neill, O. (2003) 'Some limits of informed consent'. *Journal of Medical Ethics*, 29 (1): 4–8

Partners in Care (2004) *Carers and confidentiality in mental health. Issues involved in information-sharing.* London: Royal College of Psychiatrists, at **www.rcpsych. ac.uk/campaigns/partnersincare.aspx** (accessed on 29 October 2007)

Pattison, S. (2004) 'Understanding values', in Pattison, S. and Pill, R. (eds) *Values in professional practice. Lessons for health, social care and other professionals.* Oxford: Radcliffe Medical Press

Pidgeon, N., Hood, C., Turner, B. and Gibson, R. (1992) 'Risk perception', in *Risk: analysis, perception and management. Report of a Royal Society Study Group.* London: The Royal Society

De Raeve, L. (2002) 'Trust and trustworthiness in nurse-patient relationships.' *Nursing Philosophy*, 3: 152–62

Reid, E. (2005) 'Don't be a record breaker.' *Nursing Standard*, 20 (36): 33

Robertson, J., Emerson, E., Hatton, C. and Elliott, J. *et al.* (2005) *The impact of person centred planning.* April 2005. Institute for Health Research, Lancaster University, available at **valuingpeople.gov.uk/dynamic/valuingpeople135.jsp** (accessed 15 November 2007)

Rolfe, G. (2001) *Critical reflection for nursing and the helping professions: a user's guide.* Basingstoke: Palgrave

Schermer, M. (2007) 'Nothing but the truth? On truth and deception in dementia care.' *Bioethics*, 21 (1): 13–22

Schön, D. (1987) *Educating the reflective practitioner.* London: Jossey Bass

Seedhouse, D. (1998) *Ethics: The heart of health care.* 2nd ed. Chichester: John Wiley & Sons

Seedhouse, D. and Gallagher, A. (2002) 'Undignifying institutions.' *Journal of Medical Ethics*, 28: 368–72

Sellman, D. (2006) 'The importance of being trustworthy.' *Nursing Ethics*, 13 (2): 105–15

Singer, P. (1993) *Practical ethics.* 2nd ed. Cambridge: Cambridge University Press

Skills for Care (2005) *National occupational standards for health and social care*. London: Skills for Care

Smith, C. (2005) 'Understanding trust and confidence: two paradigms and their significance for health and social care.' *Journal of Applied Philosophy*, 22 (3): 299–316

Social Care Institute for Excellence (SCIE) (2006) *Practice guide for adult services 09: 'Dignity in care'*. November 2006. London: SCIE

Thom, D.H. and Campbell, B. (1997) 'Patient-physician trust: an exploratory study.' *Journal of Family Practice*, 44, 169–76

Thompson, N. (2006) *Anti-discriminatory practice*. 4th ed. Basingstoke: Palgrave

Titterton, M. (2005) *Risk and risk taking in health and social welfare*. London: Jessica Kingsley Publishing

Trevithick, P. (2005) *Social work skills: a practice handbook*. 2nd ed. Buckingham: Open University Press.

Twelvetrees, A. (2002) *Community work*. 3rd ed. Basingstoke: Palgrave

Uslaner, E. (2001) *'Trust as a moral value.'* Paper presented at the Conference, 'Social Capital: Interdisciplinary Perspectives', University of Exeter, 15–20 September 2001

Wainwright, P. and Pattison, S. (2004) 'What can we expect of professional codes of conduct, practice and ethics?', in Pattison, S. and Pill, R. (eds) *Values in professional practice*. Abingdon: Radcliffe Publishing

Warren, M. (1973) 'On the legal and moral status of abortion.' *The Monist*, 57: 43–61. Revised version in LaFollette, H. (ed.) (1997) *Ethics in practice. An anthology*. Oxford: Blackwell

Woodbridge, K. and Fulford, K.W. (2004) *Whose values? A workbook for values-based practice in mental health care*. London: The Sainsbury Centre for Mental Health

Woogara, J. (2004) 'Patients' rights to privacy and dignity in the NHS.' *Nursing Standard*, 19 (18): 33–7

Index